Secrets of Serotonin

Secrets

of

Serotonin

The Natural Hormone That
Curbs Food and Alcohol Cravings,
Reduces Pain, and Elevates
Your Mood

Completely Revised and Updated
CAROL HART, Ph.D.

A Lynn Sonberg Book

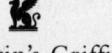

St. Martin's Griffin
New York

www.stmartins.com

Book Design by Patrice Sheridan

Library of Congress Cataloging-in-Publication Data

Hart. Carol A.
    Secrets of serotonin / The Natural Hormone That Curbs Food and Alcohol Cravings, Reduces Pain, and Elevates Your Mood / Carol Hart.—Rev. ed.
        p.   cm.
    Includes bibliographical references.
    ISBN-13: 978-0-312-37512-6
    ISBN-10: 0-312-37512-3
    1. Serotonin—Psychological aspects.   2. Serotoninergic mechanisms.   I. Title.

QP801.S4H37   2008
612.8'042—dc22

                                                                          2007048878

First Revised Edition: April 2008

10 9 8 7 6 5 4 3 2 1

Author's Note

This book is not intended to take the place of medical advice from a trained medical professional. Readers are advised to consult a physician or other qualified health professional regarding treatment of all of their health problems or before acting on any of the information or advice in this book.

Research about serotonin is ongoing and subject to conflicting interpretations. Although we have made all reasonable efforts to include the most up-to-date and accurate information in this book, there is no guarantee that what we know about this complex subject won't change with time.

Contents

Part Three: Boosting Serotonin Naturally

Foreword to the Revised Edition

The pace of research into serotonin and its roles in health and disease has roughly doubled over the past ten years, judging from the citations in the National Library of Medicine's PubMed database. The scope of that research has also broadened. Over the last decade there has been increasing research interest—and some exciting findings—regarding the important functions of serotonin *outside* the brain. On a clinical level, there is a better understanding of the role of serotonin in chronic pain conditions, including irritable bowel syndrome. On a basic science level, new research has demonstrated serotonin's role in guiding embryonic development. Quite literally, serotonin shapes us in the womb.

In recent years, scientists have identified some of the genetic factors that predispose individuals for serotonin-related vulnerabilities, such as depression and poor impulse control. These genetic factors are very common and widespread in the general population and do not in themselves produce illness. Rather, the discovery of these at-risk genetic profiles has led to an improved appreciation for how genes and environment (which includes behavior, mind-set, and lifestyle) interact to determine an individual's vulnerability to serotonin-related conditions.

It has long been recognized that most serotonin-related disorders (such as depression, migraine, irritable bowel syndrome, fibromyalgia, and bulimia) are far more common in women than in men. Ongoing research is clarifying how estrogen affects serotonin levels. Advances in brain-imaging technology have shown for the first time that *healthy women have a lower rate of serotonin synthesis in their brains compared to healthy men.*

Efforts to manipulate the serotonin system by drugs have not fared so well over the past ten years. There are growing doubts about the overall safety and effectiveness of the widely prescribed antidepressants known as selective serotonin reuptake inhibitors (which includes Prozac, Paxil, and Zoloft, among others). Nonetheless, the number of FDA-approved indications for these drugs has continued to increase. Other classes of serotonin-active medications have been withdrawn from the market or dropped from development after serious side effects were belatedly uncovered.

Recent studies have supported the natural lifestyle-based interventions described in this book. We know that the serotonin system is exquisitely responsive to eating habits, bright light exposure, sleep habits, and activity level. Relatively simple changes in how you choose your meals and organize your day can yield a substantial dividend in improved mood and energy levels. These changes are not restrictive or particularly onerous. Any increase in physical activity level—even "activities" as simple as chewing gum—can benefit serotonin system functioning. The food-mood connection is real but complex. One important component of this food-mood link has been made clear by recent studies: *Low-calorie dieting reduces brain serotonin functioning, particularly in women.* Read on—and learn how you can improve your mood, energy, bingeing, and chronic pain problems by adopting (step by easy step) a more serotonin-friendly lifestyle.

Part One

Moods,

Impulses,

Appetites,

Aches

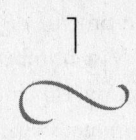

Are You Glad, Sad, or Mad?

Low moods, low energy, headaches, upset stomach, sleep problems, overeating, heavy drinking . . . we all have our patterns for responding to the stress and strain of busy schedules and lives. One person may be creative, energetic, and productive for much of the year, yet sag through most of the winter, overeating and oversleeping, like a hibernating bear or a dormant plant. Another may have daily ebbs of energy and mood that can be relieved with a fast-food fix. Someone else may cope well with work and family pressures throughout the week, then get blinding migraines as soon as the weekend comes around.

For most, these mood and energy swings and stress-response patterns aren't disabling or disturbing enough to send us to a doctor or counselor for help. We may see them as inevitable, as just the way we are. Or as an inescapable by-product of high-pressure jobs and family responsibilities. *In fact, these chronic, stress-induced problems can be minimized or even eliminated by relatively simple changes in how you eat, exercise, and organize your day.*

Have you ever noticed how often these common complaints seem to be linked? A low or anxious mood is almost always accompanied by changes in eating and sleeping patterns. Stress or changes in your eating and sleeping schedule can trigger a headache. Sometimes it isn't stress but the calendar, the weather, or the time of day that brings a sudden shift in energy, spirits, and motivation. Vast numbers of people hit their lows in the early morning or late afternoon, on cloudy days, during much of the winter, or, for women, during premenstrual days.

Although stress, weather, and season can all bring on a low mood, a headache, or an eating binge, the ultimate cause is internal and chemical. An essential natural substance called serotonin is one of the body's most powerful modulators of mood, appetite, sleep, and pain awareness. It is produced in the brains and nervous systems of humans and animals from specific nutrients in the foods we eat. Avoidable fluctuations in its availability to the brain can bring on depression, anxiety, binge eating, insomnia, headaches, and a host of other common everyday problems.

Many mood-enhancing drugs, from the antidepressant Prozac to the abused drug Ecstasy (MDMA), achieve their effects by increasing the brain's supply of serotonin. You can take nutrition and lifestyle steps to enhance your serotonin supply *without drugs* to get your mood, appetite, energy, and headache problems under control. You don't need to run ten miles a day or live on raw vegetables and skim milk. This is not a case of "the cure is worse than the disease." You can learn how to ward off your mood and energy lows by scheduling your meals and snacks and choosing mood-enhancing foods. Relaxing, low-impact exercise (for example, walking or cycling) can also help control or avoid stress reactions, such as anxiety and binge eating.

Interested? Read on! The first step is understanding why moods go up and down, and why negative moods so often bring on troubling changes in your sleeping and eating habits.

When Our Moods Just Don't Make Sense

Moods are different from emotions. We feel good when good things happen, bad when we experience something bad. We can feel glad or sad in response to a book, a movie, a newspaper article, a joke, or an insult, or something that happened to a friend. We can even feel happy or unhappy because of our thoughts, laughing at something we simply imagine, or frowning over an unpleasant memory.

But our moods often seem to be much more arbitrary, to have little to do with the good and the bad in our day-to-day lives. Moods are almost an internal weather system. A storm front rolls in out of nowhere, and suddenly we walk under a cloud, sullen, slow, and hard to please. Or irritable and anxious, getting angry or worried over trifles. When our mood shifts downward, often our emotional responses become muted or distorted as well. We don't laugh at jokes, we lose interest in normal activities and pleasures, and the little hassles and annoyances of daily life can seem not so little, maybe even unbearable.

Bad moods can come out of nowhere, but often they are surprisingly predictable. You might tend to feel bad in the mornings ("I hate to get up") or the late afternoons ("I just drag"), on overcast days, or for much of the winter. And for many people bad moods are accompanied by binge eating or drinking, or other impulse control problems, such as compulsive shopping or gambling.

The Bingeing Blues—Mood Goes Down, Eating Goes Up

Bingeing is not that wonderful dessert you can't pass up, or the four-star meal the company is paying for. Bingeing is out-of-control overeating and snacking—a compulsion to finish the box of cookies or half-gallon of ice cream when you only intended to have a bite or two. You aren't hungry, you know you've had enough, yet you can't stop. It may not be particularly good and you aren't really enjoying it, but for the minutes that you are working your mouth, chewing and swallowing, your stressed and depressed mood is miraculously better. Alcohol is also a common self-treatment for stress and anxiety. You hold yourself together all day, but need "more than a couple" to unwind in the evening.

5

Not everyone overeats or overdrinks in response to depression, anxiety, or stress. A substantial number of people lose their appetite along with their good humor, particularly if they are chronically depressed or anxious. They skip meals or push their food around their plate with little interest. However, in our "you can never be too thin" society, these individuals are less likely to complain or worry about the loss of weight they suffer during their depressed or stressed period. The association between negative mood and appetite is so common and so strong that a significant, unexplained weight loss *or* gain is considered one of the diagnostic signs and symptoms of depression.

The Stressed/Depressed Response

A sad or anxious mood can come out of nowhere, or it can be a response to stress, either a loss or setback of some kind, or more than your fair share of daily pressure. In either case, this misery usually has company. In addition to eating more or eating less, we often sleep more or less when our mood is down, and our mental and physical functioning both seem to suffer.

Negative Mood

Some people are very aware of their own moods; others don't realize that they've been irritable, uncooperative, or unresponsive until they are given that feedback. The range of feelings and behaviors that fit into the general category of "bad" or negative mood is fairly diverse: negativity about oneself or others; lack of pleasure and spontaneity; worry, anxiety, or fearfulness; obsessing about real or imaginary problems; irritability; and, of course, plain old depression.

Stressed/Depressed

Many people are more comfortable with saying that they are stressed, which sounds busy and important, than acknowledging that they might be anxious or depressed, which is still unfairly associated with weakness and mental illness. In reality, there is often not a great deal of difference between the two. Prolonged stress of any sort—physical exhaustion, physical danger, illness, emotional distress, or environmental stressors like inescapable noise—will produce signs and symptoms of depression in animals and humans. Often anxiety precedes or overlaps with the depression. Anxiety is a hyper-alert response to threats and to stress, while depression is the body's way of shutting down in the presence of intolerable strain. For some people, the stress response seems to be more sensitive, more easily triggered—for reasons that have more to do with biology than personal character.

Mood Cycles

Everyone has up days and down days, but for many of us they fall into fairly predictable patterns. Our moods, in fact, often follow the course of the sun and the moon. A great many, if not most, people will notice that their mood deteriorates over the course of a series of overcast or stormy days. Some people are very sensitive to the effects of pro-longed bad weather and suffer from what is now a well-recognized prob-lem: seasonal affective disorder (SAD). As the hours of daylight diminish in late November and December, sufferers from SAD experience chronic depression, fatigue, overeating, and oversleeping.

Less obviously, many people have a daily mood cycle that they may relate to workplace stress or unhappiness in their job. While stress can certainly contribute, there is often a clear pattern that correlates with time of day rather than with specific events. The cycle varies, but most often sufferers will feel tired and depressed in the morning, perk up toward noon, drag in the late afternoon, then feel better again after dinner.

As for the lunar cycle, mood changes and food cravings are of course very common symptoms of premenstrual syndrome (PMS), and some women can mark the exact days on the calendar when they will be trou-bled by monthly attacks of bingeing, angry or tearful moods, or mi-graine.

Sleep

Everyone has been kept awake at night or has awakened in the middle of the night because of a nagging worry; it's annoying but natural and maybe even helpful. You might find a solution to your problem or at least make peace with it by mulling it over quietly. It's much more frustrating and puzzling to be kept awake or to wake up early when there is no specific worry or problem driving your insomnia. Some people find that stressed, depressed, or negative moods will make normal sleep almost unobtainable. They may get intolerably sleepy in the middle of the day, when they need to be alert, then lie sleepless much of the night—falling asleep late or waking much too early. Insomnia is very common in a world of irregular but always busy schedules. Oversleeping is also a possible response to negative mood, and just as annoying to people who complain that they are "sleeping their life away."

Eating

Do you ever eat when you're not hungry, but because you feel bad? Few people binge because they're happy. Cravings most often hit us when we are down. Boredom alone can do it. You watch impatiently as the flight attendants work their way down the aisle passing out snack packs containing such delicacies as stale, strangely tasteless pretzels and soggy, plastic-wrapped muffins. You aren't hungry, the cuisine is hardly wonderful, but eating helps to pass the time. Depression and anxiety can make us yearn for food as a comfort and a diversion—or make eating a difficult and joyless chore. People who binge may not be depressed or anxious on a regular (chronic) basis. However, many report that their episodes of bingeing tend to occur when they are stressed or upset. Eating relieves negative feelings, at least momentarily.

Concentration/Motivation/Activity Level

During periods of anxious or depressed mood, many people report that they are unable to concentrate or that they have problems with their memory, think more slowly, and lack their normal energy and resourcefulness. A loss of motivation may be a common factor behind the drop in mental and physical performance. Lowering brain serotonin levels does impair performance on tests of memory and decision making in both animals and humans. The effect on memory is likely indirect, resulting from the serotonin system's role in modifying the activity of another neurotransmitter, acetylcholine.

Pain Awareness

Many people develop headaches, back pain, or other muscle aches when they are tense, unhappy, or angry. People with chronic pain conditions are often aware that stress will bring on another headache or exacerbate the pain of a ruptured disc, arthritis, or fibromyalgia. A few people will experience stress or depression as physical pain, and will present their family doctor with symptoms that they fear are signs of cancer, heart attack, ulcer, or some other disease. Tests will not be able to identify a physical cause of their pain. Once dismissed as hypochondriacs or attention seekers, these individuals are now known to have a distinct way of responding to stress and depression.

You may be so used to some of these familiar stressed/depressed responses that they seem logical to you. "Eating makes me feel better" or "How can I even think of eating when everything is so awful." "Of course, I can't sleep—I'm too worried" or "Sure, I sleep half the day; there's nothing worth getting up for." These explanations and rationalizations do make sense so far as they go. But they do not tell the whole story.

Serotonin: The Mood-Appetite-Pain-Sleep Modulator

Decades of research have demonstrated a very strong link between mood, sleep, appetite, and pain awareness, and serotonin, a necessary brain chemical. Normally, serotonin helps to regulate and balance these fundamental aspects of our health and well-being. Abnormalities in the amount of serotonin available to the brain have been linked with an impressive variety of disorders and everyday problems. These include:

- Depression
- Mood swings and mania
- Seasonal affective disorder (SAD)
- Premenstrual syndrome (PMS), especially moodiness and food cravings
- Anxiety
- Obsessive-compulsive behavior
- Eating disorders, particularly bulimia and binge eating, plus some forms of obesity
- Sleep disorders, especially insomnia
- Migraine and other types of headache
- Chronic abdominal pain, particularly irritable bowel syndrome (IBS)
- Heightened sensitivity to pain
- Irritability and aggression
- Poor impulse control
- Drug and alcohol abuse

These symptoms and medical conditions often show a great deal of overlap, pointing to a common underlying mechanism. For example, depression and alcoholism have been found to run in families, suggesting an inherited deficiency or instability in serotonin functioning. The same is true for migraine and depression. Studies of bulimia report that bulimics have a higher than average frequency of mood disorders (depression or anxiety) and substance abuse problems—and so do their family members. This symptom overlap is so common that it is often difficult for physicians and therapists to identify the primary or core problem with a patient who complains, for example, of poor sleep, poor appetite, and feeling keyed up or anxious.

Prozac and Company: The Serotonin-Active Drugs

Many of the drugs used to treat these common disorders are known to achieve their effects by acting on the serotonin system. Most antidepressants, including Prozac (fluoxetine), Zoloft (sertraline), and Paxil (paroxetine), increase serotonin availability or activity. So does the weight-loss drug Meridia (sibutramine), and the antimigraine medications known as the triptans (sumatriptan, rizatriptan, and many others). What's more, many serotonin-active drugs developed to treat one serotonin-deficient condition are later found to be effective for others. For example, antidepressants are often used to prevent migraine and other forms of chronic headache. They sometimes prove effective for treating binge eating, bulimia, and alcohol abuse as well, problems for which there are few medical treatments available.

Millions of people are happier, healthier, and more productive as a result of serotonin-active medication. While medication is almost always the preferred treatment for severe or chronic mood, eating, and headache disorders, many people don't want to take medication, don't need to take medication, or don't wish to continue taking it for life. Among the millions who have been prescribed Prozac or another serotonin-active drug, only a minority will need to continue taking the drug beyond a few months, or a year or two at most.

What then? How do you avoid hitting another one of life's potholes and finding yourself in another period of depression, anxiety, chronic pain, or bingeing? If you are vulnerable to the mood-lowering effects of stress or season, you will want to do all you can to minimize the toll they take on your health and happiness.

The Serotonin-Friendly Lifestyle

Fortunately, there are natural and healthy ways to help keep the brain well supplied with serotonin. An amino acid called tryptophan, which is found in a wide variety of foods, is essential for the production of serotonin by the brain and body. More attention to what you eat and when you eat it—particularly the timing of protein and carbohydrate intake—can do a lot to improve your mood at the times of day when you usually sag or drag.

Serotonin has a role in initiating movement, and movement appears to regulate serotonin in turn. The feel-good effects of a walk or other moderate exercise may be due to release of serotonin in the brain and nervous system. Experiments with animals suggest that the calming effect of chewing may well result from stimulating increased serotonin activity. Chapter 10 will suggest exercises and movement patterns you can use to enhance your body's serotonin functioning.

The effects of diet and exercise are more subtle and more moderate than those of the serotonin-active drugs. However, the simple lifestyle and nutrition changes recommended in this book have no side effects, only benefits! These natural alternatives should not be expected to re-place drugs for individuals who really need them, and you should never stop taking a prescribed medication without consulting your doctor.

If your problems with mood, eating, or headache are not severe or disabling, you can learn to recognize and avoid fluctuations in serotonin levels that affect your moods and appetite. Migraine sufferers can reduce the frequency and severity of their headaches by avoiding foods and ac-tivities known to trigger migraines as well as selecting those that will raise the brain's supply of tryptophan.

The medical and nutritional information contained in this book can benefit you if:

- You have mild-to-moderate problems with mood, food, sleep, mi-graine, or IBS and would like to know natural and healthy ap-proaches to their control.

- You are considering taking Prozac, Zoloft, Paxil, or another serotonin-active drug but want to know more about risks, benefits, and alternatives first.
- You are currently taking medication but want to know natural ways to supplement its effectiveness or to avoid a relapse when you go off your medication.
- Someone you care about suffers from one of the many medical conditions related to serotonin deficiencies.

Is It Really Serotonin?

People are complex, and so are their moods, motivations, and behavior, their personal problems, and their medical disorders. At any given moment, the one-word explanation for why you feel and act the way you do is just as likely to be "Susan," "Sunday," or "shopping" as "serotonin." But if your low mood or ill temper doesn't quite make sense to you, or if you tend to feel bad at certain times of the day, month, or year, then it is very likely that fluctuations in brain serotonin activity have a major role in how you feel.

Try answering these questions as honestly and thoughtfully as you can, to see if abnormalities or fluctuations in serotonin activity might be the key to your mood-food-sleep profile. The numbers in parenthesis after each choice are there to help you rate the severity of the symptom.

1. My moods get worse in the late fall or winter:
   _____ no (0)
   _____ mild problems (1)
   _____ moderate (2)
   _____ hard to cope (3)
   _____ severe/disabling (4)

2. I have problems with overeating in the late fall or winter:
   _____ no (0)
   _____ mild problems (1)

_____ moderate (2)
_____ hard to cope (3)
_____ severe/disabling (4)

3. I sleep more and feel tired or listless during much of the winter:
_____ no (0)
_____ mild problems (1)
_____ moderate (2)
_____ hard to cope (3)
_____ severe/disabling (4)

4. Cloudy days make me feel depressed, irritable, or low on energy:
_____ no or rarely (0)
_____ occasionally/mildly (1)
_____ frequently/moderately (2–3)
_____ almost always/strongly (4)

5. I snack when I'm not hungry or eat more than I need:
_____ rarely (0)
_____ occasionally, about once a week (1)
_____ frequently, 2–4 times a week (2–3)
_____ almost daily or daily (4)
_____ several times each day (5)

6. My moods go up and down at predictable times of day:
_____ no or rarely (0)
_____ occasionally/mildly (1)
_____ frequently/moderately (2–3)
_____ almost always/strongly (4)

7. I binge-eat or -drink more than I should:
_____ rarely or never (0)
_____ occasionally (2)
_____ frequently (4)
_____ almost daily or daily (5)

8. My eating habits change when I'm stressed or depressed:
_____ no or rarely (0)
_____ occasionally/mildly (1)
_____ frequently/moderately (2–3)
_____ almost always/strongly (4)

9. I sometimes get angry or tearful for no reason:
_____ no or rarely (0)
_____ occasionally/mildly (1)
_____ frequently/moderately (2–3)
_____ almost always/strongly (4)

10. I have food cravings and mood changes associated with PMS:
_____ no/not applicable (0)
_____ occasionally/mildly (1)
_____ frequently/moderately (2–3)
_____ almost always/strongly (4)

11. People identify me or I see myself as a moody person:
_____ no (0)
_____ yes (3)

12. My weight goes up and down a lot over the course of a year:
_____ no, or only a 1–5 pound range (0)
_____ yes, about a 5–10 pound range (1–2)
_____ yes, 10–15 pounds (3–4)
_____ yes, more than 15 pounds (5)

13. My normal sleep patterns are disrupted when I'm stressed or depressed—producing excessive sleepiness, early morning awakening, or insomnia:
_____ no or rarely (0)
_____ occasionally/mildly (1)
_____ frequently/moderately (2–3)
_____ almost always/strongly (4)

14. My sleep patterns change in the winter:
_____ no or rarely (0)
_____ occasionally/mildly (1)
_____ frequently/moderately (2–3)
_____ almost always/strongly (4)

15. I get migraines:
_____ no (0)
_____ not me, but other(s) in my family (2)
_____ yes (4)

16. I have frequent or severe headaches:
_____ no (0)
_____ yes, frequent (1–2)
_____ yes, severe (3)
_____ yes, both frequent and severe (4–5)

17. I have frequent episodes of abdominal pain or irritable bowel syndrome:
_____ no (0)
_____ yes, mildly, doesn't really bother me (1)
_____ yes, moderately, sometimes bothers me (2–3)
_____ yes, severely, has a negative impact on my life/activities (4)

If you scored yourself a 4 or 5 for several items, you should consult a health-care professional if you have not already done so. In addition to medication, behavioral therapy and stress reduction training can be very helpful in gaining understanding and control over these (seemingly) diverse mood, food, sleep, and pain problems. If any of your symptoms are severe or disabling, you should not expect that the health- and nutrition-oriented information provided in this book will offer you a cure. The serotonin-friendly lifestyle *can* supplement and enhance the effectiveness of medication or behavioral approaches, and hopefully give you a good basis for keeping your mood, food, or pain problems under control in the future, if you are not one of those who require long-term medication use.

If you scored yourself 1 to 3 on several questions, that is a strong indicator of mild-to-moderate serotonin system deficiencies that can be addressed by nutritional and other lifestyle modifications. This book will help you understand your symptoms and spot the times and circumstances that put you at risk for mood drops, headache or abdominal pain attacks, insomnia, binge eating, or other serotonin-related problems. You will learn how to choose meals, snacks, and daily activities that will ward off the low points and the bad days—helping you maximize the time you spend at your peak of energy, productivity, and good spirits. No restrictive diets or elaborate exercise regimens will be required. Instead, the recommendations offered will guide you to select a wholesome variety of good foods and a level of physical activity that suits your health and preferences.

Quite likely, there is no one who can say "I never feel anxious, angry, or sad for no reason," "I never have trouble sleeping at night and staying alert during the day," *and* "I never binge or overeat." Our schedules and lifestyles conspire against it. More and more of us sit at a desk all day doing jobs that require a sustained level of concentration and effort that we just may not be able to give all day, every day. Overrefined sweet and fattening foods are always readily available to soothe anxiety and tension. There is caffeine to keep us up during the day, alcohol to bring us back down at night. We frequently disrupt our sleep schedule for shift-work, deadlines, or late-night entertainment. Slight inherited serotonin deficiencies can be greatly aggravated by a serotonin-*un*friendly lifestyle—the kind most of us practice. Even if your moods, sleeping, and eating are only occasionally thrown out of kilter by your schedule, this book can help you avoid serotonin-related problems in how you work, eat, relax, and play.

If your mood-food-sleep-pain symptoms trouble you, if you would like to get better understanding of and control over them, read on! This book will help you by explaining how and why:

- Mood and impulse control problems arise from biochemical deficiencies, not weakness or lack of will power.

- Abnormalities in brain serotonin are believed to be a major underlying cause of both everyday and severe problems with migraine, IBS, moodiness, and bingeing.
- Biochemistry is not destiny! You can gain control over your mood-food problems through medication, lifestyle changes, or a combination of the two.
- Diet and physical activity impact the brain's production of serotonin.
- Exercise and repetitive physical movements can boost serotonin production.
- Small, simple changes in what you eat and when you eat can help stabilize your serotonin levels naturally.
- Serotonin-active drugs are often effective in treating anxiety, depression, headaches, IBS, and eating disorders—how they work, what they can do, and their risks and side effects.

Healthy foods and regular exercise will be recommended, but you don't have to diet or do strenuous workouts in order to achieve a more serotonin-friendly lifestyle. You only need to pay attention to the timing of your meals and snacks and to their relative protein and carbohydrate content. A simple Food-Mood-Activity Journal will help you prove to yourself that the balance and timing of your protein and carbohydrate intake do make a difference in how you feel, and so do certain types of physical activity. You may find, in fact, that your mood and motivation improve to the level that you are able to pay more attention to your health and fitness—getting more exercise and eating from hunger rather than stress. And that would be the best of all possible outcomes!

2

How One Little Molecule Can Do So Much

If you are the kind of person who likes to ask "Why?" "How does it work?" "Who says so?" and "Can you prove it?" this chapter will give you some answers. Question number one undoubtedly is, "What *is* serotonin?"

Serotonin is a neurotransmitter, a specialized molecule that allows nerve cells to communicate and interact with each other. Without neurotransmitters we would be unable to think, perceive, move, or even live. Serotonin also does double duty in the cardiovascular and gastrointestinal systems. It helps regulate the expansion and contraction of blood vessels and the function of platelets, the blood cells that cause blood to coagulate and close a wound. It controls or modulates many normal aspects of food digestion *and* indigestion, including nausea and vomiting.

About thirty neurotransmitters have been identified, some of them very specialized and others with a range of job duties in different parts of the brain and nervous system. Along with acetylcholine, dopamine, and norepinephrine, serotonin is among the most significant in terms of the number and importance of the functions it helps carry out. In fact, the nerve cells that release and receive serotonin extend throughout the brain

19

and down to the spinal cord. This serotonin system is the largest single system in the brain, influencing a broad range of basic functions from movement to mood.

All these different neurotransmitters work together in processing our thoughts, sensory perceptions, decisions, and actions. Although the cortex, the wrinkled gray matter of the brain, is in charge of making all the "executive" decisions, the brain seems to function as a sort of democracy. Many different centers in the brain take part in processing basic information that helps to determine when we eat and sleep, whether we feel pain, whether our energy, mood, and motivation levels are up or down. The multiple neurotransmitters and the different processing centers provide a system of checks and balances. It's safe to assume that more than one neurotransmitter and one group of nerve cells are involved in carrying out each of the brain's many complex tasks. This way, one can pitch in and try to cover when another is not doing its job.

One of serotonin's major roles is to modulate or control the effects of other neurotransmitters. Basically, this means it can influence the relative importance or priority of the messages sent by other neurotransmitters, giving them a green, red, or yellow light. This helps to explain why serotonin can have such pervasive effects on our mood and behavior, yet does not act alone. In the words of Thomas Carew, a Yale University researcher, "Serotonin is only one of the molecules in the orchestra. But rather than being the trumpet or the cello player, it's the band leader who choreographs the output of the brain."

The Lock and the Key to the Mystery

Like people, the body's organs and cells have to communicate with each other in order to function and to survive. As their language, they use a great variety of specialized chemical messengers that include the neurotransmitters and the hormones. Serotonin and other messenger molecules pass signals from one cell to another by interacting with special gatekeeper molecules called receptors. It is a lock-and-key system, in which each messenger molecule can unlock and activate only a specific receptor type. When a messenger molecule attaches to the proper receptor, the receptor triggers a series of responses within the cell, which may then release its own messengers to pass the information on to yet other cells. Serotonin is known to unlock at least fifteen different receptor subtypes, each thought to have a distinct role in influencing some aspect of mood, functioning, and behavior.

Many common diseases are caused or aggravated by too much or too little activity by one or more of the body's many messenger molecules. This is true of conditions as varied as breast cancer, Parkinson's disease, and hay fever. Drugs to treat these disorders often achieve their effects by mimicking the shape of a messenger molecule and tricking the receptor into responding. Others block the receptor and prevent it from interacting with its usual messenger molecule. Still others affect some part of the process by which the body produces the messenger molecule and then breaks it down after it is used. For example, Prozac, Zoloft, and Paxil are "serotonin reuptake inhibitors," also referred to as SRIs or SSRIs. Normally, serotonin is pumped back into the nerve cell that released it after it is used once. These drugs interrupt that process so that more serotonin is available to reach the target receptors. Serotonin-active drugs for mood or eating disorders generally act to *increase* the availability or activity of serotonin in the brain.

All of this is test tube–based theory. Does it really explain what happens when the drug reaches our bodies and brains? Probably, but as we shall see, there is some reason to doubt. Some "weak" serotonin reuptake inhibitors are just as good at relieving depression as more powerful SSRIs. An antidepressant called tianeptine used in France actually has the opposite effect of Prozac—it increases reuptake or removal of serotonin—yet is quite effective in relieving depression. Perhaps all we can say with any certainty is that these drugs "tweak" an ailing serotonin system, stimulating it to normalize its functioning. Unfortunately, the power of that tweak can also cause changes in other brain signaling systems, producing imbalances and side effects.

How Do We Know?

As you may have guessed, there is no precise way to know what a chemical is doing, in real time, within the brain of a living person. Sophisticated techniques to study the brain's chemistry in action are now being used in animals, but these are too invasive to be used in human volunteers. Our current understanding of serotonin is largely based on animal studies, on autopsies of disease and suicide victims, and on more limited studies of human volunteers with serotonin-related conditions. Many people are uncomfortable with animal experimentation, yet neurotransmitter research is one of the areas in which it provides invaluable help in understanding the brain and treating its disorders.

Autopsies of people provide important information, especially in understanding the role of serotonin in suicide and Alzheimer's disease. Also, clinical studies involving patients can obtain useful data by analyzing the level of serotonin metabolite (its chemical breakdown product) in the spinal fluid, or (less invasively) by assessing the presence of other secondhand indicators of serotonin activity in blood samples. Some studies give a serotonin-active treatment to volunteers and then use verbal or written questionnaires to find out the impact on their mood or appetite. All these studies have limitations, but taken together they provide an impressive body of evidence to show serotonin's importance to our daily functioning. Over the last decade, specialized noninvasive brain scans have been developed that can track activity in serotonin brain centers or even detect levels of serotonin synthesis. Although not widely available, this sophisticated technology has begun to yield new insights (as well as confirmation of the older research) into the functioning of serotonin in health and in disease.

Serotonin Does Not Act Alone

We mentioned the fact that the brain puts more than one chemical signaling system in charge of each aspect of mood, behavior, movement, and mental activity. Norepinephrine, also called noradrenaline, is believed to have a secondary role in setting our moods. In the brain's "wiring circuits," the norepinephrine system seems to run fairly parallel to the serotonin system, suggesting some different and some overlapping functions. A few drugs that act mainly on the norepinephrine system are quite effective in treating depression. In the realm of mood, norepinephrine is an "activating" chemical. It is released in response to stimulants such as coffee and amphetamines, in response to stress, and in anxiety attacks. In contrast, serotonin activity is believed to promote a feeling of calm and well-being.

Serotonin's Source

Where does serotonin come from? It is synthesized in different parts of the brain and body, where it can be stored or released. The most important raw ingredient is an amino acid called tryptophan. Amino acids are the building blocks of protein, and tryptophan is found in all high-protein foods, such as dairy products, eggs, meat, and fish. (Vegetarians also have many good sources for tryptophan, including seeds, nuts, and a number of vegetables.) When these foods are digested, their amino acids, including tryptophan, enter the bloodstream and are carried to tissues that will use them to synthesize the body's own proteins and other essential molecules, including serotonin.

Some dramatic experiments with animals and human volunteers have demonstrated how dependent we are on dietary tryptophan for our moods. Animals that are deprived of tryptophan will show noticeable behavior changes, becoming much more aggressive. In one study, healthy men were given one of two amino acid beverages to drink as their meal. One mixture contained no tryptophan; the other contained tryptophan as well as other dietary amino acids. It was a double-blind "is-it-Coke-or-Pepsi" type of experiment. Neither the volunteers nor the researchers knew which cocktail was which until the study was over. The results? The men who drank the mixture without tryptophan had noticeable deteriorations in mood on that day. On the day they were given the full, balanced amino acid mixture, their moods did not change in any significant way.

This tryptophan depletion experiment has been repeated by multiple researchers studying behavior and serotonin in different populations of healthy individuals and patients. Only people whose depression assessment scores suggest they never had a bad day in their lives seem immune to the sobering and mood-lowering effects of the tryptophan-free beverage. (In case you are curious, it tastes really nasty, even with a generous squirt of chocolate syrup.) This relatively low-tech experiment provides the best evidence for the important role of serotonin in fundamental mood and behavior. Briefly, tryptophan depletion results in:

- a modest mood drop in healthy, normal-mood women that is greater than the drop seen in healthy, normal-mood men
- a complete, if temporary, recurrence of depression symptoms in patients under treatment with antidepressants
- a mood drop in people whose depression scores are normal but borderline
- a mood drop in normal-mood people who have a family history of depression; this mood drop is substantially greater than in a matched group of volunteers who had no family history of depression
- a worsening of symptoms (binge-eating and irritability) in patients with active bulimia, and a recurrence of bulimic symptoms in recovered patients
- anger or anxiety in patients with autism
- increased irritability in PMS

- either no change or increased anxiety in patients with generalized anxiety disorder
- increased compulsive behavior in obsessive-compulsive disorder

So will a cheeseburger make you cheerful? Should you load up on protein in order to feel better? Although it is true that tryptophan comes from protein, not from fats or carbohydrates, you actually need a well-timed carbohydrate meal or snack in order to increase the amount of tryptophan reaching your brain. How this works—and how you can use it for your benefit—will be explained later, in chapter 8.

You may be wondering why people take an antidepressant drug to increase serotonin availability to the brain. Why not just take serotonin itself? The answer is that serotonin cannot pass from the bloodstream into the brain. The brain controls and limits the number of substances passing into it, somewhat like a nation that guards its borders, allowing only a certain number of "foreigners" to enter. This "border check" is called the blood-brain barrier. The blood vessels that carry oxygen and nutrients to the brain have less permeable walls than the vessels that service the rest of the body. This is a safety feature. If we drink, eat, or inhale something toxic, our brains have a better chance of continuing to function. The brain, of course, welcomes the amino acids it needs to function, but they can pass out of the blood into the brain only very slowly and in relatively small numbers.

It should be mentioned that only 10 percent of the body's supply of serotonin is found in the brain. The rest is produced in the gastrointestinal tract, where it has many functions, some not yet fully understood.

Serotonin in Sickness and in Health

Health is more subtle and complex than disease, and much less well understood. The list of disorders in which serotonin abnormalities are believed to be a major factor keeps expanding. It includes mania, depression, anxiety, personality disorders, suicide, impulsive acts of violence and aggression, obsessive-compulsive behavior, some types of sexual problems, alcoholism, compulsive gambling and other forms of addiction, eating disorders, sleep disturbances, and perhaps schizophrenia and Alzheimer's disease. In addition, serotonin abnormalities underlie migraine, cluster headache, and other forms of chronic headache, as well as fibromyalgia and chronic abdominal pain complaints such as irritable bowel syndrome. It is also thought to contribute to some cardiovascular conditions, including Raynaud's disease and hypertension.

Because the list is so long and includes such extremes of behavior, from mild anxiety to murderous aggression, some researchers have suggested that a better way of understanding serotonin in health and disease is to focus on its normal roles in regulating mood, impulse, and appetite. When serotonin functioning is thrown out of balance, the impact can be felt in any number of ways. Depending on genetics and environment, that imbalance might make itself known as migraine or abdominal pain attacks, bingeing, anxiety, obsessive-compulsive behavior, depression, or out-of-control impulsiveness.

Mood

Low moods and low serotonin go together, a finding that has been confirmed in study after study for several decades. Most of these studies are based on depressed or anxious patients, people who are significantly ill and have sought medical treatment. Yet all the evidence suggests that the normal role for serotonin is to balance and adjust our normal mood shifts, somewhat like the bass-treble knob on your stereo. It has a role in *habituation,* the process in which the brain learns that a particular recurring sensation (such as background noise) is not all that important and should be ignored. When the serotonin system is functioning normally, it helps us keep a steady frame of mind amid all the things happening to us and around us. It helps us "tune out" the unimportant stuff and respond in a balanced way to the things that do matter.

We would like to be happy and carefree all the time, but there are times when it is appropriate to be sad, cautious, or worried. Serotonin helps establish that response and our corresponding activity and impulse level. Twenty thousand years ago, it may have been appropriate to be subdued and listless all winter long, or when the weather didn't permit us to hunt or gather food. It isn't now, yet many of us still respond powerfully to season, weather, and time of day. Or react too sensitively to stress and to other triggers in our overcivilized lives. Our serotonin system becomes less active in response to environmental influences, like stress, irregular schedules, or bad weather, and we then get the mood-food-pain symptoms as a result. However, you can take steps to counterbalance the impact of environmental factors and daily stresses on the serotonin system. Some food and lifestyle choices will depress serotonin functioning, while others will enhance it.

Motivation

Motivation is difficult to define, but we all know when we have it, or when we don't. Being down for any reason seems to rob us of our motivation. We know we should go out, call a friend, get busy, do something. We know that activity and exercise makes us feel better, but we can't shake the low mood and the lack of motivation. We stay in front of the TV or in bed, maybe with a bag of cookies to comfort us.

In animals, serotonin has been shown to have an important role in initiating movement. Serotonin seems to be the switch regulating movement versus sensory perception. Have you ever noticed how a cat or dog will freeze to listen to a sound or to watch a bird or squirrel? At that moment when the animal holds still and uses its senses, serotonin activity drops. When the animal moves again, serotonin activity returns. We often think of ourselves as doing "ten things at once," but we humans also tend to freeze when we want to pay attention to something important.

An anxious person or animal often becomes hyperalert to sights and sounds, perhaps forcing a low serotonin even lower! Reduced serotonin activity could be the common link between depressed mood and the apathy, the lack of interest in moving and doing, that so often comes over us when we are low. Some people, when they are seriously depressed, will have a physical slowing of speech, movement, and responsiveness that can be quite noticeable to others around them.

Impulse Control and Aggression

Serotonin seems to have a very important role in inhibiting impulsive behavior and action. We generally think of inhibition as an undesirable trait. However, without inhibitions, we would quickly ruin relationships, lose jobs, and quite possibly land in jail! We would certainly eat and drink and act on sexual or aggressive impulses with no thought for the consequences.

Of course, none of us are born knowing how to behave ourselves. We learn to control our impulses in response to rewards and punishments handed out by parents, siblings, teachers, and playmates. Although *normal* impulse control is a complex, learned behavior, *abnormal* impulse control is now believed to be related to poor serotonin system functioning. Children and adolescents who have a history of poor impulse control—excessive aggressiveness, setting fires, or other antisocial behavior—have been found to have abnormally low serotonin levels. Extreme forms of impulsive or aggressive behavior—violence against others or self (suicide, self-mutilation)—also show a strong link with low serotonin availability in the brain. In the last few years research has suggested that common variations in specific serotonin system genes (particularly SERT, the serotonin transporter gene) lead to an increased risk of poor impulse control manifested as suicidal behavior, childhood violence, or more severe and antisocial forms of attention deficit disorder. Human behavior is far too complex to be predicted by a few gene variations, however. Many different genes, in concert with such important influences as education, upbringing, stress level, and alcohol use, are presumed to be involved in an inability to stifle dangerous aggressive impulses.

On an everyday, law-abiding level (no guns, knives, or fists), aggression is difficult to define and quantify. We often think of it as a wholly negative quality, but in fact appropriate expression of aggression is an essential survival and success skill. Because of the difficulty of defining and studying complex character traits, it is not known whether healthy levels of aggressiveness and assertiveness are also regulated by serotonin, yet many researchers believe this is a reasonable assumption. Recent research has linked a common genetic variation in a specific serotonin receptor (5-HT_{2A}) with an impulsive, go-ahead-and-damn-the-consequences style of decision making on a standard psychological test.

Serotonin Shapes Us in the Womb

Although until very recently, research on serotonin has focused on its presence in the brain and nervous system, it has long been known that the fetus develops receptors for serotonin at a very early stage—before the brain and nervous system are formed. Scientists therefore reasoned that serotonin must be important for directing crucial stages of embryonic growth and development. Studies in animals indicate that serotonin directs normal development of the face and skull, the nervous system, the cardiovascular system, and the gastrointestinal system. Since the embryo at this early stage has no ability to synthesize serotonin, normal development depends upon the mother's own serotonin, which passes through the placenta to the fetus. This research is very current (the report establishing the role of maternal serotonin appeared in the January 2, 2007, issue of *Proceedings of the National Academy of Sciences*). It raises the hypothesis—to be explored in future studies—that abnormalities in the mother's blood serotonin (too much, too little, or too many fluctuations) might explain some serotonin-related disorders (such as autism) that seem to run in families but for which no underlying gene defects have as yet been identified.

Appetite

On an everyday level, serotonin controls appetite. The sight, smell, or expectation of food stimulates serotonin release in the hypothalamus, a part of the brain known to regulate feeding and sleep. As eating begins, serotonin continues to rise, until it registers in the hypothalamus as the experience of satisfaction or satiety. That "I'm full" feeling in your stomach actually comes from your brain!

Even though a half dozen other brain chemicals are known to be involved in regulating appetite and food intake, the influence of serotonin is impressive. Experiments have shown that if you increase serotonin availability or activity, you will tend to reduce food consumption. Decreasing serotonin system activity will tend to increase food consumption.

Alcohol and Nicotine Cravings

Alcohol may be our oldest medicinal and recreational drug. Millions of people "self-medicate" anxiety or depression with a drink. How many old movies have you watched in which Humphrey Bogart, or some other poker-faced tough guy, poured a few belts or got downright drunk in order to deal with fear, loss, or confusion? You don't have to be an alcoholic to have problems with alcohol. You may be drinking more than you would like, more than you consider healthy, yet find that you crave alcohol to smooth or lift your mood in the same way that other people crave chocolate or potato chips. In both cases, low serotonin availability may excite the craving. Drinking alcohol temporarily raises serotonin levels, then lowers them. As a treatment for feeling low, booze actually brings us even lower.

The evidence linking smoking to serotonin is more limited. The brain has specific receptors that interact with nicotine and are responsible for the symptoms of craving and withdrawal that make quitting so difficult for smokers. It has been speculated that serotonin may make a contribution as well, through its role in controlling craving and impulse. In experiments with animals, nicotine will increase serotonin activity in some parts of the brain. Also, serotonin-active treatments will decrease the frequency with which rats "give themselves" nicotine. No one has yet trained a rat to hold a cigarette and puff, but once they are given nicotine, they are hooked. They will run through a maze, work a treadmill, or push a lever over and over—in effect, they'll "walk a mile for a Camel"—to get another dose! A particular type of serotonin receptor is thought to have a role in reinforcing the stimulating and gratifying effects of stimulants such as caffeine and nicotine.

As most smokers, ex-smokers, and their significant others know all too well, the toughest part of quitting is dealing with the mood and appetite changes they experience. People trying to quit cold turkey will become very irritable, and either sudden or slow nicotine withdrawal will increase appetite and food cravings. Virtually every ex-smoker will gain a few pounds, and for many people this is the biggest deterrent to stopping. The fact that the mood-and-food symptoms of smokers attempting to quit match those of serotonin-deficient conditions suggests that nicotine does interact with the serotonin system in complex, not-fully-understood ways. If you are a smoker who would like to quit but have not been able to do so, following the dietary guidelines in part three may help make your mood and food symptoms more tolerable. You should expect a short-term weight gain, however, and postpone any dieting until after you have your moods and eating habits back to normal.

Drug Abuse

If "low" serotonin makes you feel "low," will "high" serotonin make you feel "high"? Well, in a way, yes, but it's temporary, dangerous, and illegal! Several abused drugs are known to act on the serotonin system. MDMA (Ecstasy) is a very powerful serotonin-active drug. Although it may have effects on other brain chemistry systems, it produces its feelings of euphoria and tranquility primarily through its action on serotonin receptors. Several hallucinogenic drugs, including LSD and psilocybin, resemble the serotonin molecule so closely that they are also believed to produce their psychedelic effects by acting on serotonin receptors.

Much evidence links serotonin abnormalities to alcoholism and other substance abuse. Substance abusers do have lower levels of serotonin activity, and serotonin-active drugs decrease alcohol and drug abuse both in humans and in rats—who are not so different from us after all! However, the degree of improvement varies greatly from individual to individual. It is thought that low serotonin may contribute to substance abuse through serotonin's effects on impulse control, food and fluid intake, and on mood. Anxiety, depression, and poor impulse control are often part of the profile and the problems underlying alcohol and drug abuse.

Heart and Blood Flow

Serotonin is found in platelets, the blood cells that clump together to close wounds, and it helps them do this important job. It also has complex roles in regulating blood flow to the brain, heart, and gastrointestinal tract. It regulates blood vessel elasticity and can act as either a vasodilator (causing vessels to expand) or a vasoconstrictor (causing vessels to narrow), depending on where and when it is released.

Because of its complex action in controlling blood flow and blood pressure, serotonin abnormalities are also thought to have a role in a number of other cardiovascular conditions, including some forms of hypertension (high blood pressure). These include peripheral vascular diseases, which are circulatory problems involving the blood vessels in the extremities, the hands and feet, and sometimes the lower legs as well. One of these, Raynaud's disease, is characterized by numbness, discoloration, and pain in the fingers or toes on exposure to cold. Although it is called a disease, it usually does not require treatment, though it can sometimes interfere with activities such as winter sports or swimming in cold water. As mentioned, serotonin appears to be involved in some forms of hypertension (high blood pressure). Ketanserin, a serotonin-active drug that acts to lower serotonin availability, has been used to lower blood pressure.

Migraine and Other Chronic Headache

Serotonin system abnormalities are believed to play a major role in causing migraine headache, cluster headache, and possibly tension headache. In persons who are prone to migraine, there is a defect in a specific type of serotonin receptor that normally causes blood vessels to constrict. Because of this defect, different irritating triggers can cause vessels supplying blood to the brain to expand (dilate), putting pressure on surrounding tissues and causing pain and tenderness. Antidepressants are often but not always effective in preventing these headaches. Some people will find that their migraines will miraculously go away if they take Prozac, while others will get the worst migraines they have ever had.

In general, low brain serotonin levels are associated with increased sensitivity to pain, and chronic pain sufferers appear to have reduced serotonin functioning. Serotonin is known to have an effect on pain awareness, in part by controlling the release of a pain-signaling brain chemical called substance P.

Gastrointestinal Effects

Contractions of the abdominal smooth muscles are involved in normal digestion and in nausea and vomiting. Serotonin causes the smooth muscle of the gut to contract when it is released by the nerves supplying the muscle. Under normal conditions, serotonin regulates the regular waves of intestinal contractions that move food through the digestive tract. Underactivity or overactivity of the gut serotonin system can produce the pain and other symptoms of irritable bowel syndrome (IBS). Nausea and vomiting are largely under the control of serotonin centers in the brain stem. Several drugs that block a specific serotonin receptor ($5\text{-}HT_3$) have offered considerable benefit to cancer patients by minimizing the nausea and vomiting associated with chemotherapy. These so-called setron drugs, which include Zofran (ondansetron), Kytril (granisetron), Aloxi (palonosetron), and Anzemet (dolasetron), tend to produce constipation, and some of them have been used for diarrhea-predominant IBS. Lotronex (alosetron) was approved for this indication, withdrawn for a serious side effect, but then remarketed with restrictions.

Sleep-Wake Cycle

Serotonin activity in the brain stem is highest while we are wide awake and is absent during REM sleep, the period of sleep in which we are actively dreaming (REM stands for "rapid eye movement," another distinguishing feature of this sleep stage). During REM sleep, when serotonin function is close to nil, we are temporarily paralyzed, since serotonin is necessary for initiating voluntary muscle movement. This is an important safety feature provided by serotonin, since without it we might attempt to act out our dreams, hurting ourselves and possibly others. As we wake up in the morning, serotonin activity increases, providing us with get-up-and-go, literally and figuratively. Since sleep and mood are both regulated by serotonin, mood problems tend to bring sleep problems with them, either insomnia or oversleeping. People with low serotonin have been found to spend less time in non-REM sleep, the longest part of the normal sleep cycle. Restless leg syndrome, the annoying muscle spasms and restlessness that interfere with sleep, has also been related to low serotonin functioning.

During the night, serotonin is metabolized by the brain to create melatonin, a very important hormone for regulating sleep. Between them serotonin and melatonin regulate the sleep-wake cycle, keeping us alert during the daylight hours and allowing us to sleep at night. Chapter 3 will explain in greater detail the relationship between serotonin and melatonin and what is now understood about their importance in ensuring normal sleeping patterns.

Mental Functioning

During periods of depression and anxiety, people do poorly on tests of mental functioning, such as memory and concentration. These results are paralleled in experiments with animals who are given a serotonin-depleting drug or diet. It is not clear whether serotonin has a direct role in mental functioning. It may be that a decline in motivation and attention, rather than in actual mental ability, is the explanation for why low mood states and poor mental functioning seem to go together. On a practical level, it hardly matters. When our mood is depressed, so is our mental performance.

Another neurotransmitter called acetylcholine is generally believed to have the leading role in memory. However, serotonin may take the "best supporting role" nomination, with a strong secondary influence on our ability to learn and remember. Animals can still learn and use memory when given treatments that deplete *either* acetylcholine *or* serotonin levels. However, a treatment that deprives them of both neurotransmitters will result in profound loss of memory and learning skills.

Serotonin functioning decreases in old age and much more severely with Alzheimer's disease. Autopsies have shown a drop in the number of serotonin receptors in Alzheimer's sufferers. At this point, it is believed that low serotonin functioning may be responsible for the mood and behavior problems of people with Alzheimer's disease, who are often anxious and depressed and may become very aggressive and impulsive in the later stages of the disease. Antidepressants have been reported effective in improving mood and behavior for these patients, potentially a very great benefit for them and for their caregivers.

More Women Than Men—Why?

Most, but not quite all, of the serotonin-related conditions that will be discussed in the following chapters occur at a much higher frequency in women than in men:

- Eating disorders: 90 percent of those affected are women
- Fibromyalgia: 90 percent of sufferers are women
- Migraine: 70 percent of sufferers are women
- Seasonal affective disorder: two to three times more common in women

- Dysthymia (borderline depression): two to three times more common in women
- Major depression: two times more common in women
- Generalized anxiety disorder: two times more common in women
- Agoraphobia: two to four times more common in women
- Irritable bowel syndrome: two times more common in women

Why? The prime suspect would obviously be estrogen. For some of these conditions—migraine and depression are good examples—the increased incidence in women is clearly linked to estrogen cycling and to reproduction. Before puberty and after menopause, females have no greater vulnerability to depression and migraine than males of the same age. For affected women, symptoms are often worse when estrogen levels drop in the days before their period—bringing on the negative mood symptoms of premenstrual syndrome (PMS) or a menstrual migraine attack. Mood and migraine problems may go away entirely in the second and third trimesters of pregnancy (when estrogen levels are high), to return with a vengeance after childbirth (when estrogen levels drop abruptly).

How? This question is more complex and the answer is not entirely clear. Estrogen has been shown in study after study to affect serotonin synthesis and activity in the brain, but the effects are not uniform throughout the brain or under differing experimental conditions. Much of the past research has been based on studying the effects of giving estrogen back to female rats that have had their ovaries removed. This research indicates that estrogen has a general stimulatory effect on serotonin activity. However, experiments of this type cannot tell us much about the effects of natural estrogen cycling in females with their ovaries intact. Highly sensitive brain chemistry imaging techniques are now beginning to provide some answers. One such study utilizing a form of Positron Emission Tomography (PET) scan found that the average rate of *brain serotonin synthesis* is 52 percent higher in healthy men than in healthy women, but with a substantial variation from one individual to another.

When the serotonin-specific PET scan was repeated after the study participants had consumed a tryptophan-free mix of amino acids, the women had a more drastic lowering of brain serotonin levels than the men. Previous studies had found that healthy women reported a bigger mood drop, compared to healthy men, in the tryptophan depletion experiment. Now we know why.

This research brings us closer to understanding why there is a higher risk for depression, migraine, and other serotonin-linked disorders for women compared to men. Under normal conditions, brain serotonin *levels* appear to be roughly similar between men and women (again with large individual variations). It is the rate of serotonin *synthesis* that varies so dramatically between men and women. Since stress has been shown to deplete brain serotonin levels in animal studies, this lower rate of synthesis may be an explanation for why women are more prone to stress- and serotonin-related problems, like depression, bulimia, and migraine.

These biological differences seem to be true for the females of many species. But it is unlikely to be the case that estrogen (or estrogen cycling) has only negative effects on serotonin functioning. Evolution is a slow but very efficient process for eliminating harmful traits that impair survival. Somehow the low estrogen–low serotonin link must have had a positive, or at least a neutral, effect on a female's health and her ability to raise healthy offspring.

It is often the case that genetically linked disorders that affect a substantial number of people actually provided a survival benefit in a closer-to-nature environment. The classic example is the gene responsible for sickle-shaped red blood cells. Children who inherit the gene from both parents will have sickle-cell disease, a frequently debilitating and potentially fatal condition. However, inheriting just one copy of the gene (producing sickle-shaped red blood cells) greatly increased the odds of surviving malaria, a disease that still kills one million children each year worldwide.

There are theories (right now they are only theories) as to why disorders like depression and migraine might have once had a survival advantage, particularly for women. These will be discussed, at least briefly, in later chapters. These ideas are worth discussing because they offer a more positive way of looking at serotonin-related problems. At some point in the distant past, the tendencies or vulnerabilities that now cause you suffering might have been very useful adaptations to a harsher environment. Binge eating when you are stressed or worried might have been a good idea, long ago, when the biggest worries and stresses had to do with impending food shortages. In the traditional rural life of subsistence farmers, for example, the rhythm of life was feast or famine, not feast and feast (with a snack or two in between), as it is now. As another example, being timid or anxious isn't very glamorous, but a cautious, expect-the-worse-and-be-prepared mind-set might have helped your ancestors stay out of trouble in a rough and dangerous world.

From this perspective, *it is not you* (with your migraines or binge eating or anxiety or seasonal affective disorder) *but the artificial environment in which you live that is defective.* Physical inactivity, too little exposure to natural daylight, irregular sleep habits, and poor nutrition can all have a negative impact on serotonin functioning in persons with an inherited vulnerability. Part three will guide you in identifying and changing the aspects of your daily life that are out of harmony with your natural serotonin system functioning.

Can You Have Too Much of Such a Good Thing?

If too little brain serotonin is linked with depression, anxiety, bulimia, bingeing, insomnia, out-of-control aggression, migraine, and alcoholism, then do you want to have as much serotonin in your system as possible? If we are talking about natural approaches to increasing brain serotonin system activity, then the short answer is yes for people who are troubled by negative moods, bingeing, or the other symptoms of low serotonin.

However, an overdose or inappropriate combination of serotonin-active drugs can be quite serious, even deadly.

Serotonin Syndrome

Serotonin syndrome is an emergency condition caused by an over-dose or accumulation of serotonin-active drugs. The symptoms are variable but may include confusion, agitation, heavy sweating, shivering, high fever, loss of coordination, and muscle spasms or weakness. It is not easily diagnosed, particularly when the sufferer's confusion and agitation make it difficult to identify the underlying cause. Treatment involves administering fluids, plus medication to control blood pressure, which is usually high. The syndrome typically resolves within a few days, but it has been fatal in a few cases. Once considered to be a rare complication of treatment (linked to a little-used class of drugs known as monoamine oxidase inhibitors or MAOIs), the incidence of serotonin syndrome has been increasing over the last decade with the growing number of serotonin-active drugs and supplements on the market.

Serotonin syndrome can occur when someone is taking multiple serotonin-active drugs for different medical conditions. In particular, serotonin syndrome has been reported in individuals taking one of the triptan drugs for migraine along with an SSRI or SNRI, serotonin-norepinephrine reuptake inhibitor, antidepressant. This is a serious concern, since people who are biologically prone to either condition are also at risk for the other. Moreover, headache specialists sometimes prescribe an antidepressant for headache prevention in addition to triptan medications for headache relief. It really is not clear how great (or small) the risk is. As of July 2006, the Food and Drug Administration had received reports of twenty-seven cases, which would represent a tiny fraction of all the people using these two common classes of medication, but there may be many other cases that go unreported or even undiagnosed. Mild cases, characterized by sweating, tremors, and agitation, might simply be mistaken for anxiety.

Since the Food and Drug Administration issued an advisory for this risk in July of 2006, physicians *should* be aware of the potential for serotonin syndrome and avoid prescribing antimigraine triptans with antidepressants unless truly necessary. If, however, you are seeing one specialist for headaches and another for a mood disorder, it is important to make sure all your health-care providers know what prescriptions you are using, even if you only take a triptan occasionally. The following drugs were included in the FDA advisory bulletin:

Antidepressants	Triptans
SSRI Antidepressants	
Celexa (citalopram)	Amerge (naratriptan)
Luvox (fluvoxamine)	Axert (almotriptan)
Lexapro (escitalopram)	Frova (frovatriptan)
Paxil (paroxetine)	Imitrex (sumatriptan)
Prozac (fluoxetine)	Maxalt (rizatriptan)
Symbyax	Relpax (eletriptan)
(olanzapine/fluoxetine)	
Zoloft (sertraline)	Zomig (zolmitriptan)
SNRI Antidepressants	
Cymbalta (duloxetine)	
Effexor (venlafaxine)	

Healthy individuals taking an SSRI or SNRI antidepressant only (no other serotonin-active medications) at prescribed doses are not at risk of serotonin syndrome, but the syndrome has occurred in frail elderly persons who have been prescribed too high a dosage for their age, weight, and general health. In particular, accidental overdosing of the antidepressant Effexor has produced serotonin syndrome; reportedly, the syndrome occurs in roughly 15 percent of all SSNI overdoses. So, if you are taking one of these drugs, it is really crucial to track doses carefully, never risking an extra dose because you can't remember whether you've already taken your meds, or because you're feeling particularly low (an extra dose won't help). The abused drug MDMA (Ecstasy) can cause serotonin syndrome at doses normally taken by abusers. Combining serotonin-active drugs with supplements such as Saint-John's-wort or 5-HTP (5-hydroxytryptophan) can also trigger the syndrome. These supplements should not be taken along with a serotonin-active drug without your doctor's knowledge and supervision.

The triggering factors and true incidence of serotonin syndrome are still not known. If you are taking serotonin-active medications or supplements and are experiencing times when you are inexplicably sweaty and shaky, with your heart racing, particularly if these panic-like symptoms are accompanied by dilated pupils and muscle spasms, it's a possibility to discuss with your doctor.

Too Thin—Too Much Serotonin?

Some researchers believe that self-starvation (anorexia nervosa) may be related to elevated serotonin in certain parts of the brain. Several studies have reported that anorexics have higher levels of serotonin metabolite in their spinal fluid, implying a higher level of brain serotonin activity, both during their fasting and purging episodes and after long-term weight restoration. Since serotonin produces a feeling of fullness after eating, individuals with higher serotonin activity might have too little appetite or feel full after eating very little. A role for some type of serotonin abnormality is likely, since sufferers are often depressed, anxious, and obsessive, which are all serotonin-associated problems.

Low serotonin can make you feel low, and high serotonin can make you feel high—which in fact is how the illegal drug Ecstasy works. But life is much more complicated than that, and serotonin serves many different functions in the brain and body. High serotonin in specific parts of the brain can make you feel anxious; in other parts it will make you vomit. For many serotonin-related conditions, all we know for certain is that serotonin system functioning is suboptimal, either underresponsive or overresponsive to the events in our lives, skewing our moods and impulses in an unhappy or unhealthy direction.

Autism—Too Much Serotonin?

Over the past few years, evidence has been accumulating to suggest that abnormalities in blood serotonin levels (derived from the gut, not from the brain) may be an underlying cause of at least some forms of autism. Individuals with autism frequently (but not always) have abnormally high levels of serotonin in the blood. Abnormal serotonin levels have also been found in the blood of parents of autistic children even when the parents have no symptoms of autism. As noted above, serotonin from the mother's blood is an important modulator of normal fetal development. One current theory proposes that fluctuations in maternal serotonin levels may have subtle effects on brain development. This is an area of great research interest but (currently) very little certainty. *If* maternal blood serotonin levels do influence the risk of autism, it is not even clear whether the increased risk results from too high, too low, or too variable levels of serotonin in the blood—or whether those abnormalities are primarily triggered by genetic factors (can't be helped) or lifestyle factors (can be helped). This may be yet another area in which a healthy lifestyle during pregnancy—exercise, well-balanced meals, and good sleep habits—has subtle positive benefits for mother and child.

Chemistry + Events = Mood + Behavior

It is currently fashionable to see our personalities, our diseases, and our problems as more or less determined by genes and hormones. To a large extent, this is because researchers are discovering so much so fast about the chemistry of life and disease. But we should never forget that the other half of the equation—our environment, our lifestyles, and our experiences—has an even greater influence. There certainly are some inherited tendencies that are absolute. Blue-eyed parents will produce blue-eyed children. If a mother or father has Huntington's disease, the children who inherit the gene will inevitably develop the disease. For the most part, though, our genes and our hormones only direct our tendencies.

Serotonin abnormalities do seem to be inherited since, more often than not, people with migraine, mood disorders, alcoholism, or other serotonin-related conditions will have other affected family members. In 2003, an important study by an international team of researchers reported that differences in SERT (a crucial serotonin system gene) were linked to increased vulnerability to depression following major life stresses. (By way of background, the SERT gene makes the serotonin transporter that takes up excess serotonin and removes it from the system. The SSRI antidepressants—Prozac, Zoloft, and others—target this serotonin transporter to block its action and so allow more serotonin to stay in the system.) The two common versions of the SERT gene differ in length, and the short version of the gene is the one associated with increased vulnerability to depression after stress. We inherit one copy of the gene from each parent, so people with two short versions have the highest risk of depression, those with one short and one long have an intermediate risk, and the lucky ones with two long versions have a tendency to roll with life's punches.

Tendency is the operative word here. The 2003 report on the influence of the SERT gene did not find that people with the short copies of the gene were "naturally" more depressed. In the absence of a stressful life event (such as illness, unemployment, or a failed relationship), the type of SERT gene, short or long, made no difference in the risk of depression. Rather, people who have the short version of the gene seem less resilient, less able to cope and recover from a major setback. Even so, *less able* does not mean incapable. Young adults who had had four or more recent stresses had about a 40 percent risk of serious depression if they had the short version of the gene, compared to a 20 percent risk for those with the long version. People with only the long version of the gene weren't immune to depression; it is just that depression wasn't linked to stressful life events in this group of people.

The SERT gene is only one of many that affect serotonin system functioning and potentially influence mood and behavior. Other gene profiles might make an individual more prone to depression in response to chronic hassles, perceived failures, social slights, cloudy days, premenstrual tension, or all the other factors, big and small, that can affect our mood.

How these individual differences in our genetic endowment play out depends very much upon our daily experiences and our environment. We certainly can't control everything that happens to us. But choosing a lifestyle that acts to stabilize and enhance serotonin functioning can make food, mood, and pain symptoms more manageable and less frequent.

3

Serotonin-Sunny by Day, Melatonin-Mellow by Night

Melatonin is a hormone produced in the brain that is necessary for normal sleep. It is available as an over-the-counter supplement and was once wildly hyped as a cure for just about everything, including cancer and aging. Much of the initial enthusiasm for melatonin as either a treatment for serious illness or an enhancement of normal good health has evaporated after two decades' worth of interesting, but inconclusive, studies. There is reasonably good evidence for its effectiveness in minimizing jet lag and relieving insomnia. It may also be beneficial for seasonal affective disorder (SAD) and some forms of depression, but here the evidence is weaker. Because each person's daily rhythms of melatonin production are unique, the optimal timing and dose of supplemental melatonin is difficult to determine, even by experts.

If you are troubled by insomnia, there are alternatives that are even more "natural" than melatonin. *Your body makes its own melatonin from serotonin.* Nutrition and lifestyle changes that will boost and stabilize your serotonin system will also have a positive effect on your natural supply of melatonin.

Melatonin is synthesized by a tiny pea-sized organ deep inside the brain called the pineal gland, which is well supplied with serotonin.

Along with serotonin, melatonin appears to be one of the master hormones that help to regulate the twenty-four-hour patterns in the body's functioning, called the circadian cycle. Together, melatonin and serotonin take part in regulating the sleep-wake cycle and daily body temperature changes, along with seasonal variations in hormone secretion.

Melatonin production is triggered by darkness and turned off by light striking the eye. In animals (and presumably people) the production of melatonin can turn on and off almost as immediately as flipping a light switch. During the night the amount of melatonin circulating in the body increases by a factor of ten, and serotonin release drops markedly at the same time. Once the pineal gland starts pumping out melatonin, drowsiness begins to bring on sleep. With luck, it is lights out and melatonin on for six to eight hours, when daylight or the alarm clock will tell your brain that it's time to move into the serotonin part of the circadian cycle.

The Serotonin-Melatonin Cycle

For some people, the serotonin-melatonin cycle goes out of sync all too readily. This happens, unavoidably but temporarily, when we fly across several time zones and experience jet lag. Our body's clock is still timed to the twenty-four-hour cycle of our starting point, and may take as long as a week to synchronize with the time shift, depending on how many times zones we have crossed. Melatonin production continues to follow the familiar cycle of your home time zone, particularly if you are spending most of your time indoors and inactive at your travel destination. Without sufficient exposure to natural light, particularly at dawn and dusk, the pineal gland lacks the most important cue it needs to readjust its schedule of melatonin production. Sleep, mood, and appetite may all suffer, and chronic headache sufferers often get attacks when travel rearranges their daily schedule.

Many people have a mild, semiannual "time lag" experience without leaving home. When the clocks are changed from daylight savings time to standard and back again, the one-hour change can bring on serotonin-related symptoms in susceptible individuals. Sufferers from SAD sometimes get their first symptoms when the clocks are turned back in the fall. Curiously, cluster headache sufferers often get a reduction in headache attacks at the "fall back" and "spring forward" time, as discussed in chapter 5.

Often work and play throw our biological clocks out of order as well. Shift workers have great difficulty adapting their internal clocks to their work schedule, and both their sleep and their work performance suffer as a result. Taking melatonin supplements before going to bed has been reported to help in obtaining sleep. However, studies have indicated that work performance does not improve, perhaps because the pineal gland is still producing melatonin during the nighttime, which is the shift worker's daytime.

A Matter of Timing: The Phase-Shift Theory

The body's clock is an ancient timepiece—even plants and cockroaches are tuned to the cycles of the day and the year. The internal clock (located in the hypothalamus) used by higher animals, including humans, was probably well evolved by the time of the dinosaurs. It doesn't need batteries, it doesn't need winding, yet it keeps time remarkably well, provided it gets essential environmental cues from the passage of the sun across the sky and the changes in light intensity over the course of the day and of the year. The body must have a timekeeping mechanism to determine essential daily cycles in temperature, food and water consumption, sleep-wake, and activity level, as well as monthly and annual cycles of fertility and growth—just to name a few of the more obvious ones. Every organ in the body appears to follow a twenty-four-hour rhythm in its growth, functioning, and repair. If an animal is kept in darkness, its melatonin synthesis and other biochemical processes will continue to cycle on a roughly twenty-four-hour basis, but will gradually become disassociated from the natural day-night cycle outside the laboratory. Usually, the clock tends to run fast if it is not reset regularly by morning light. Human beings who manipulate their exposure to light and dark with artificial lighting are subject to phase shifts in which the rhythm of the internal clock becomes uncoupled from the rhythm of the sun. Hormonal factors, such as estrogen, can trigger a phase shift, and this shift of the biological clock is thought to have a role in symptoms of PMS. In fact, women with premenstrual sadness or anxiety have signs of altered nighttime melatonin activity.

When we deliberately substitute artificial light for daylight and nightfall, we also break the link between the biological clock and natural day. Chronic and occasional insomnia may be worsened by the fact that reliance on artificial light for daytime and evening activities can throw the inner clock out of phase, even for people who keep to a fairly regular schedule. When this happens, the normal cycle of daytime serotonin activity and nighttime melatonin production is shifted forward or back so that we become sleepy during the day or wakeful at night. Night owl insomnia (delayed sleep phase insomnia), discussed below, is one of the more common consequences. This phase-shift theory has also been used to explain some forms of depression, including the winter blues, or SAD.

Melatonin and Serotonin in Sickness and Health

∽

Sleep-Wake

Between them serotonin and melatonin may be the master regulators of daytime alertness and voluntary movement versus nighttime sleep and benign paralysis, which is the inability to move while in deep sleep that keeps us from acting out our dreams. Disorders of sleep can come from any number of sources, but abnormalities in the melatonin-serotonin cycle are implicated in a number of sleep problems, ranging from ordinary insomnia to sleepwalking. Serotonin's relationship to sleep is complex and involves interactions with other neurotransmitter systems as well, in particular the acetylcholine (cholinergic) and norepinephrine (noradrenergic) receptor systems that were briefly described in chapter 2.

There is good evidence to show that serotonin receptors in the brain stem have a crucial regulatory role in maintaining wakefulness. Serotonin-active treatments can increase or decrease wakefulness, and serotonin-deficient disorders such as depression often include either insomnia or oversleeping. It is thought that one of serotonin's basic functions is to modify or suppress vigilance or an overaroused state of being. We become vigilant or hyperalert during acute stress, a state that can lead to either depression or anxiety. Because serotonin is a mood modulator that serves to calm or reduce tension, increasing serotonin availability could have some mood-related effects on permitting sleep, in addition to allowing production of melatonin, which directly affects sleeps.

Melatonin can cross the blood-brain barrier (explained in chapter 2), while serotonin, which is a larger molecule, cannot. This is part of the reason why you can't "take" serotonin as a treatment for sleeping problems or other serotonin-related disorders. To increase serotonin, you must take a drug that interacts with the brain's serotonin system or use dietary measures to increase the amount of tryptophan reaching the brain. The supplement L-tryptophan (which the brain can convert to serotonin) was widely used as a sleeping aid in the 1980s before it was taken off the U.S. market after a tainted shipment resulted in serious illness and death.

To date, melatonin appears to be moderately effective and safe as an occasional treatment for insomnia. For this purpose, a recommendation in general use is to take 2-3 milligrams (mg) one to two hours before bedtime; however, doses as low as 0.5 mg may be effective. Timing of the melatonin dose is very important when it is being used to reset the body's clock to prevent jet lag or to treat phase-shift insomnia. Otherwise, the melatonin may bring on sleep without solving related problems of daytime drowsiness. It is most likely to be beneficial for specific types of insomnia—for example, delayed sleep phase insomnia—if prescribed by an experienced sleep specialist. However, as we'll see, there is a safer and more natural treatment—increased exposure to natural daylight to reset the body's clock—that should be tried first for chronic insomnia before you consider taking a powerful hormone on a regular basis.

To treat jet lag, melatonin doses from 0.5 to 5.0 mg have been used in studies. The strategy used is to begin taking the melatonin supplement in your home time zone at the time you would go to bed in your destination time zone. Then continue taking the supplement at bedtime for several days after your arrival in your new time zone. Although some studies have reported good results with this regimen, others have not. Success seems to depend on the criteria used in the study. As a jet lag remedy, melatonin may reduce daytime sleepiness without improving late-night wakefulness. Many business travelers who trot the globe from meeting to meeting, conference to conference, believe they do better by following their normal sleep-wake schedule if they are away from home only for a few days at a time, even if this means getting up at 4 A.M. and going to bed by 8 P.M. Vacationers may do best by running up a sleep debt on arrival (this assumes they will not be doing anything requiring good concentration, like driving a car), then getting enough daylight exposure (particularly early morning light) to reset the internal clock. Active vacationers (hikers, cyclists, etc.) are less likely to be inconvenienced by jet lag, since daytime activity helps reset the clock in addition to making it easier to sleep at night.

Core Body Temperature

Every day the body's temperature rises during the day to peak around evening, then drops during the night for a low point in the early A.M. hours. The peak release of melatonin during sleep coincides with the nighttime drop in the body's core temperature. As discussed in chapter 2, an overdose or interaction of serotonin-active drugs can cause a serotonin syndrome that includes a high fever, suggesting that serotonin turns up the body thermostat during the day.

Heart and Blood Vessels

Melatonin is believed to have anticoagulant properties, meaning it reduces the likelihood of clots forming that might result in stroke or heart attack. Serotonin, on the other hand, helps in the body's defensive maneuvers (clotting and inflammation) in the event of an injury to a blood vessel. It is present in platelets, the sticky blood cells that clot together to close wounds and prevent excessive bleeding. Melatonin may have an indirect link to regulating blood pressure. Serotonin has a better understood effect on blood pressure through its ability to regulate blood vessel elasticity (dilation and constriction).

Immune System

The immune system, like so many of the body's functions, follows a daily cycle of activity in which melatonin appears to have a role. During the night, the cycle of melatonin production parallels increased nocturnal activity of infection-fighting white cells. When the immune system is stressed by disease or cancer, melatonin production generally increases, suggesting that it is a component of the body's self-defense response. Have you ever gotten sick after air travel and blamed the man two rows back who kept sniffling and blowing his nose? In fact, planes have ventilation systems as good as or better than office buildings or other indoor spaces. Colds, flus, and other ailments associated with travel may be brought on by the disruption in the normal circadian rhythms of the immune system. Stress, depression, and other interference with the circadian rhythms (jet lag, shift work, skipping sleep) are all associated with reduced immune function and increased infections.

Fertility and Sexuality

In animals, a wintertime surge in melatonin production acts to keep the female from going into heat and becoming pregnant during the seasons of the year when offspring are less likely to survive. In the 1990s there was research interest in Europe in developing a new and possibly safer birth control pill that would combine melatonin with progestin. A clinical trial of this combination reported promising results in 1992, but no further studies appear to have been done, possibly due to lack of funding to investigate a nonpatentable (and therefore less profitable) treatment. In laboratory experiments, serotonin seems to be important to moderating or inhibiting sexual behavior. Depending upon which area of the brain is tried, injections of serotonin or serotonin-active drugs can increase or decrease mating behavior in male and female rats. In humans, serotonin deficiencies have been found in individuals with histories of sexual misconduct (criminal or psychiatric)—not surprisingly, given serotonin's importance for impulse control.

Hormones and Cancer Control

Melatonin released by the pineal gland acts on the pituitary gland, the master gland of the body's hormonal system. It stimulates or suppresses the release of a number of hormones that affect growth, metabolism, and reproductive cycles, including growth hormone, estrogen, and testosterone.

It has long been known that the growth of cancer of the breast is fueled or promoted by estrogen, and prostate cancer likewise grows in response to testosterone. Because melatonin evidently has a role in controlling the release of the sex hormones, it is thought that melatonin may have value for preventing or treating breast cancer and possibly prostate cancer as well. In the laboratory, researchers have grown colonies of breast cancer cells and experimented with exposing them to melatonin. Cancer cells that were rich in estrogen receptors grew much more slowly when treated with melatonin than untreated cells. Melatonin suppressed growth by about 25 to 50 percent in these cancer cell colonies. The fewer estrogen receptors found on the cancer cells, the less effect melatonin had on slowing cancer growth. It had no effect on tumors that lacked estrogen receptors.

Melanoma is another hormonally sensitive cancer. In laboratory experiments with cultured melanoma cells, melatonin has been found to suppress the growth of the cancer. Some other evidence suggests that melatonin production may increase as a cancer fighting measure. In a number of types of cancer, a higher melatonin level correlated with improved prognosis.

This sounds very promising, but human cancer, alas!, is much more complex than a laboratory Petri dish of cultured cells. Studies to date have failed to demonstrate that melatonin supplements can change the course of any of these cancers.

Antioxidant Effects

In addition to its beneficial effects on hormonal factors that fuel cancer growth, melatonin has also been identified as a free radical scavenger, or antioxidant. As you probably know, one prominent theory suggests cancer and aging are linked to cell damage caused by free radicals. These are unstable molecules within the body that react with other molecules and render them unstable. If a free radical attacks the DNA in a cell, it can damage the cell so that it can no longer function. Another, more sinister possibility is that a free radical might cause the DNA to change so that the cell divides to create a mutant, cancerous cell. A free radical scavenger or antioxidant agent such as melatonin is basically one that can safely react with a free radical, rendering it harmless to the body's tissue. While it is certainly true that free radicals have the potential to damage cells, the theory that free radicals cause cancer and aging is, at this point, only a theory. There are other rival explanations for the aging process for which the evidence is just as persuasive.

Free radicals are unavoidable. They are released as an inevitable by-product of the body's metabolic processes, and you are making more free radicals with every breath you take. Some of the enthusiasm for taking antioxidant supplements has faded since beta-carotene, one of the most popular supplements, was found to be ineffective at best in preventing or controlling disease in two large, well-designed studies. This does not mean that antioxidants produced by the body or obtained naturally from the diet might not have helpful, even vital, contributions in protecting the body from free radical damage. It is reassuring that the foods richest in antioxidants are the very ones your mother said to eat: citrus fruits, carrots, tomatoes, broccoli, and cabbage—and the list goes on to include most fruits, vegetables and whole grains. In addition to all their other benefits, these are also foods beneficial for boosting the brain's production of serotonin.

Aging

Mysteriously, the brain's supply of both serotonin and melatonin declines with age, a fact that may help to explain why the elderly often suffer from insomnia and have an increased risk of depression. In one experiment, researchers placed the pineal glands of young mice in the brains of old ones and achieved a 25 percent increase in expected lifespan. Another group of investigators who added melatonin to laboratory animals' drinking water reported a 20 percent increase in lifespan. On the basis of these experiments, it has been theorized that melatonin might have antiaging effects, and that increasing melatonin to compensate for the natural decline in its production by the pineal gland might prolong life. Before you accept this theory and rush out for a six-month supply of supplemental melatonin, you should reflect that the body's production of many hormones declines with age, and these natural declines may in fact be protective against heart attack or cancer. Remember the claims made for the health-enhancing, life-extending effects of hormone replacement therapy in postmenopausal women—until the Women's Health Initiative study found that hormone replacement increased the rates of breast cancer, heart attacks, and strokes.

Mood

Some studies have reported low melatonin levels in people suffering from depression, and also in alcoholics, even when abstinent. It is not clear whether a melatonin deficiency might cause depression or other mood-related problems. It may be the case that an underlying serotonin deficiency causes both the low mood and the lower melatonin production.

Following the phase-shift theory, some researchers have suggested that the chronic or cyclical mood problems result from a disturbance in the time-keeping function of the hypothalamus, which is shifted forward so that the individual has reduced energy during the day and sleep problems during the night. Bright light exposure in the evening has been used to treat PMS symptoms, with a beneficial effect credited to increased or normalized melatonin-serotonin cycling.

Melatonin has been used to treat depression, but its effectiveness is not proven. Increasing melatonin levels through supplements has sometimes *increased* brain serotonin levels and sometimes *decreased* them. Potentially, melatonin supplements could free more serotonin for use in daytime mood and behavior control. It's also possible that overuse of melatonin supplements can disrupt the natural balance in serotonin-melatonin production or result in dependency on the supplements. Nutrition and exercise remain the best, first-line approaches to managing symptoms related to serotonin and melatonin activity.

Melatonin is thought to play a role in seasonal affective disorder—either through excess melatonin secretion, producing a persistent lackluster drowsiness, or badly timed melatonin secretion, meaning that people with winter blues are not properly in cycle with the long winter nights and short days. However, results of one recent study (discussed in chapter 4) suggest that it is actually the people with clinical SAD who are in natural harmony with the seasons. They appear to have a longer duration of nighttime melatonin secretion during the winter months—a relic of our animal past that the rest of us have lost. The National Institute of Mental Health is currently conducting a trial to see if partial suppression of melatonin will relieve the symptoms of SAD. Somewhat confusingly, melatonin is also used to treat SAD, although there is disagreement about its efficacy. In this context, it is given in the afternoon, in small doses, to induce a corrective phase shift.

There is general agreement that the duration and timing of melatonin and of bright light exposure are both involved in SAD, both as causes and cures. However, there is still little certainty about the precise mechanisms. The person who is prone to winter blues may be especially sensitive to the effects of light or may have a circadian clock that adjusts poorly to changing light exposure (or that fluctuates in the absence of strong environmental lighting cues). For some of us, problems with getting up before sunrise or on an overcast day may be a natural body rhythm—the lack of a strong trigger to turn off melatonin production. But try telling that to your boss! SAD is reported to worsen with age, and sometimes the seasonal mood problems become year-round depression, suggesting that natural, age-related declines in serotonin and melatonin levels could be a factor.

More About Serotonin, Melatonin, and Sleep

Poor sleep may be the nation's number one undertreated health problem. An estimated 40 million Americans have chronic sleep disorders, while another 20 to 30 million have occasional sleep problems. In one survey, just over half the population said that they got less sleep than they needed. Inadequate sleep is thought to be a factor in well over a quarter million car accidents per year. Poor sleep can be a passing reflection of short-term stress, anxiety, or depression, or it can result from some deficiency in the serotonin-melatonin wake-sleep cycle. A few sleep disorders appear to have a strong link to serotonin or melatonin abnormalities.

Sleep Apnea

Once thought to be relatively unusual, a disorder called sleep apnea is known to be an often undetected cause of poor sleep and daytime fatigue. The sufferer has changes in the airways during sleep in which muscle tone weakens and the airway is partially blocked. A stop in breathing occurs, and can recur every few minutes throughout the night. Loud snoring, with frequent gasps and sputters as the sleeper struggles for air, are telltale signs. Often a spouse or roommate is more conscious of the problem than the sufferer, who may not be aware that he or she is waking up for seconds at a time gasping for air over and over again. Sleep apnea is most common among middle-aged or older men who are seriously overweight. Estimates of its prevalence range from 5 to 10 percent, but the vast majority of sufferers have never been diagnosed. Studies suggest that deficiencies in serotonin activity in the brain stem may be responsible. Serotonin has an important role in maintaining muscle control and tone via the nerves supplying the airway. Serotonin-active drugs, such as mirtazapine, have been studied for sleep apnea, but so far there is no strong evidence to support their use.

Narcolepsy

In narcolepsy, deep sleep can strike at any moment—while a person is driving a car, during a meeting, sitting at a desk, or even standing up. A related condition, cataplexy, involves a sudden loss of muscle tone while awake during moments of emotional excitement or sometimes of stress. Both conditions seem to involve mistimed brain activity that involves serotonin system nerves in the brain stem. Normally, these nerves have a significant role in maintaining the benign cataplexy or temporary paralysis that occurs during REM sleep.

Sleep Paralysis

Did you ever wake up in the night and find yourself unable to move and struggling for breath? This frightening but harmless condition is so common that many different cultures have a name and a myth to explain it. Folklore usually calls on the idea of a witch or ghost who sits on your chest or grips your throat. This momentary paralysis can suddenly vanish if the sufferer is touched or called by name. Sleep paralysis is common for narcoleptics, but people with no other sleep abnormalities may have an occasional episode. Estimates of the incidence of sleep paralysis range all the way from 5 to 60 percent. Like daytime cataplexy, this nighttime sleep paralysis is thought to involve some timing problems in the sleep-wake cycle, in which the paralysis that is normal during REM sleep (when serotonin activity is minimal) occurs during waking. Sleep paralysis can occur whenever the normal sleep–wake cycle is disturbed, such as after a period of sleep deprivation or as a result of jet lag.

Sundowning

In addition to sleeping less and more fitfully, the infirm elderly are subject to a phenomenon called sundowning, in which they will become confused, agitated, and disoriented around sunset or in the evening, particularly in the fall and winter. They may also wake up in the night and wander around with similar symptoms of disorientation and confusion. In many cases, the elderly person who might be able to live at home with a spouse or adult child is institutionalized because dealing with the sundowning effects is so difficult. One study found that sundowning was the major reason for placing an elderly relative in a nursing facility. The low level of lighting in many houses and nursing homes is believed to be a factor in sundowning, which may involve an impaired or disordered circadian cycle. Use of light therapy is reported to help both sundowning and insomnia in the elderly. A 1997 Dutch study found that a midday fitness program was effective in normalizing circadian rhythms for ten healthy men in their early seventies. For the healthy elderly, as for younger people, regular exercise can improve daytime alertness as well as sleep quality.

Restless Legs Syndrome

With sleep paralysis you wake up to find yourself unable to move. Sufferers from restless legs syndrome have just the opposite problem. They are unable to stop moving. They will have an uncontrollable impulse to move their legs that may make it difficult to fall asleep or may actually wake them up repeatedly during the night. Serotonin abnormalities are thought to have a role; however, antidepressants can make the restlessness worse. A related sleep disorder called nocturnal myoclonus is more likely to disturb the sleep of the sufferer's bed partner. In this condition, the muscle contractions and restlessness are generally not noticed by the sufferer, who is only momentarily awakened by them.

Night Owl Insomnia

Otherwise known as delayed sleep phase insomnia, this is the most common form of out-of-phase sleep-wake cycle. People with night owl insomnia find it nearly impossible to fall asleep before 2 A.M. (some will be awake and alert until dawn), but will then have a normal six or eight hours of good rest, provided their schedule doesn't require an earlier rising. Adolescents with late-night study and socializing habits and shift workers are among those most likely to have delayed sleep phase insomnia. It may not be a problem until they have to make a transition to the standard 9-to-5 schedule, then find they are functioning (or not functioning) on three hours of sleep. They cannot simply reset their alarm clock to get on the normal schedule. Their circadian cycle—which controls serotonin, melatonin, other hormones, body temperature and other basic metabolic functions—needs to be reset, too.

Although obviously there are lifestyle factors involved in night owl insomnia (the worker on the night shift and the student doing all-nighters), it tends to run in families, so there may be genetic risk factors as well. In studies involving volunteers kept in constant dim light, without clocks or watches and without the cues of day and night, there are large variations from person to person in how well the internal clock keeps time.

Night owl insomnia is best managed by morning light exposure—ideally, two hours of bright light between 6 and 8 A.M. However, since this is the middle of the night for the insomniac, many people find it very difficult to comply with the recommendation. Any level of early-morning light exposure (including working under bright lights or near a window) may be a help. Sleeping in on the weekend, although very tempting, perpetuates the phase-shift problem, since the individual is missing the morning light exposure needed to reset the internal clock. Additionally, there is some evidence to suggest that people with delayed sleep phase insomnia are particularly sensitive to the melatonin-suppressing effects of light in the evening. Bright lights in the morning, dim lights at night, and outdoor exercise during the day are helpful (but not magical) in getting the internal clock reset to a more normal and natural cycle.

Compared to morning light exposure, melatonin in the evening is less effective in resynchronizing the sleep-wake cycle, but it may be more convenient for people who cannot schedule that hour or so of bright light into their mornings. The timing and dose are far from standardized, and many different dosing regimens have been tried. Higher doses produce effects similar to standard sedative drugs. They bring on sleep but may not correct the underlying problem with the timing of the sleep-wake cycle. Taking melatonin shortly before bed, the usual recommendation for treating ordinary insomnia, will not treat the out-of-sync problem of delayed sleep phase. Instead, the melatonin should be taken about five hours before the usual bedtime, in order to gradually push the onset of drowsiness forward to a more reasonable hour. In some studies, the delayed sleep phase insomnia returned within a few days after melatonin treatment was stopped. It is important to avoid operating machinery while taking melatonin, since even small doses can produce drowsiness.

Early-Bird Insomnia

Insomnia can also result from an advance phase shift, although it is much less common. In this instance, irresistible drowsiness strikes in the early evening, 6 P.M. to 9 P.M., with a very early wakeup time of 2 A.M. to 5 A.M. It is more common with age, and many elderly people who complain of an early awakening may be phase advanced. Melatonin is not a convenient treatment for advanced sleep phase insomnia, since in this setting it needs to be taken daily during the night or very early morning, usually producing daytime drowsiness. Simply forcing oneself to stay up later will not reset the clock; the evening drowsiness and the early morning awakening will keep recurring. To delay the sleep period of an individual who has advanced sleep phase insomnia, bright light exposure in the first half of the evening (roughly between 7 P.M. and 9 P.M.) is necessary. This treatment is delivered by a light therapy panel or box, which is also the most effective treatment for seasonal affective disorder, and is discussed in more detail in chapter 4.

More Melatonin Naturally—See the Light!

If you are reading carefully, you may be puzzled by the different prescriptions for using melatonin and bright light as treatments for out-of-phase forms of insomnia. That's because melatonin and bright light therapy have opposing effects on resetting the circadian clock. Either melatonin in the evening *or* morning light exposure will correct advanced phase insomnia, resetting the clock to an earlier bedtime. Either melatonin in the early-morning hours *or* evening light therapy will correct delayed phase insomnia, resetting the clock to a later bedtime. Some people with severe symptoms may do best with a combination of melatonin and light exposure, delivered at opposing points on the day-night, serotonin-melatonin cycle. Although melatonin is reasonably effective, properly timed bright light therapy produces a stronger readjustment in the internal clock, making it the treatment of choice for SAD and sleep phase insomnias.

Bright light therapy has also been used in combination with antidepressants for nonseasonal depression. There is a demonstrated dose response pattern, and any exposure to bright indoor or outdoor light seems to have a generally stimulating effect, helpful to people who have problems with low mood and low energy. A recent study found that increased daytime bright light exposure increased the peak amount of melatonin secreted during sleep. In short, brighter days (and darker nights) may be generally effective in improving both sleep quality and daytime alertness.

If you have symptoms of SAD, sleep problems, or bad weather moods, increasing your exposure to bright light is a reasonable and safe approach, provided you protect yourself from sunburn resulting from prolonged direct sun exposure. Indoors, bright broad-spectrum white lights are also recommended for daytime use. For obtaining more natural daylight effects, shielded full-spectrum lights can be tried in the rooms you most use. The full-spectrum fluorescent tubes and modified bulbs are more expensive, but they are also more energy efficient and can last three to ten times longer than ordinary fluorescent and incandescent lighting. These lights may also be helpful for headache sufferers who are sensitive to glaring and flickering lights.

The Melatonin-Serotonin Balance

Increasing serotonin through lifestyle and dietary measures apparently also increases nighttime melatonin release. Taking Prozac or related SSRI antidepressants does not, and many individuals suffer from insomnia as a side effect. These drugs act to decrease total sleep time and REM sleep. The relationship between melatonin supplements and serotonin activity is both complex and unclear and needs more research—another reason to be cautious about the use of melatonin. Some forms of depression and SAD may respond to appropriate and well-timed doses of a melatonin supplement. For many people, the only obvious consequence will be a slight increase in fatigue. Consider melatonin a drug, and don't try it as a therapy for SAD, depression, or chronic sleeping problems, unless under a doctor's supervision. There is no proof that it prevents cancer or slows aging.

If you do want to boost your immune system, lower your blood pressure, sleep better, reduce your risk of cancer, and improve your energy level, there is only one proven safe and effective approach that does it all: a sensible diet that stresses complex carbohydrates, vegetables, and fruit, plus regular, preferably daily, exercise. Since a healthy, high carbohydrate diet and regular exercise are also effective in raising brain serotonin activity and melatonin production, you do get it all in one package. At the same time, you avoid the risk of boosting levels of one "miracle" hormone at the cost of all the other health-promoting substances the body manufactures and uses.

Part Two

~

Serotonin Out of Sync

4

Feeling Low: Depression, SAD, PMS

Low serotonin, low mood. The partnership of serotonin and mood has been confirmed in study after study. The extent to which we depend on serotonin to sustain our moods has been shown in the tryptophan depletion experiments described briefly in chapter 2.

A series of tryptophan depletion studies in depressed patients have been reported by researcher Pedro Delgado and colleagues. For these studies, the research team prepared two different amino acid concoctions, one with all the dietary amino acids found in milk, and another that differed only in lacking tryptophan, the amino acid that the body requires to make serotonin. For the volunteers drinking the second concoction, blood levels of tryptophan fell dramatically. The experiments were double-blind and crossover—meaning that neither the researchers nor the volunteers knew who was getting which mixture, and each volunteer was tested with each mixture on different days.

This experiment was first done with healthy men who had no history of mood disorders. On the day of drinking the no-tryptophan mixture, these men reported experiencing a noticeable drop in mood. In another study, volunteers who had been treated for depression in the past were given the no-tryptophan mixture, which produced a striking but brief return of symptoms in fourteen of twenty-one participants. For example, three hours after drinking the tryptophan-depleted potion, a woman widowed four years earlier began to weep and grieve as if her husband's death had just happened. Late the next day, after normal food consumption, her mood abruptly lifted and she was back to normal. Many other studies that have measured markers of serotonin activity in the blood and spinal fluid have indicated that people suffering from depression have reduced serotonin system activity.

Low mood, low serotonin. Much evidence suggests that the reverse is also true: Low mood leads to low serotonin system activity. Stress is known to lower blood tryptophan levels in animals, presumably resulting in reduced serotonin synthesis in the brain. When something truly terrible happens and we feel appropriately depressed, our brain evidently responds to the emotional blow by reducing serotonin activity. There may be types of depression that involve changes in other brain neurotransmitter systems, such as the norepinephrine system. The fact that serotonin-active drugs are effective for post-traumatic stress disorder would suggest that our brains and bodies may respond to personal losses and other environmental stressors by lowering serotonin system activity.

This fact raises a dilemma for counselors and therapists. If someone has suffered a terrible loss and has symptoms of severe depression, should you offer to treat them with antidepressants? When does normal grieving become abnormal depression? The textbook rule is that symptoms that seem out of proportion to the loss, or that persist for more than three months after a major life stress, should be evaluated for depression. Our thoughts and feelings—our minds—can influence or even determine the chemical balances of the physical brain. The most powerful antidepressants will not make us cheerful if we have a major loss or stress to work through.

The Depressed Response

Think of depression as a normal biological process. Suppose you are traveling for business or pleasure, a snowstorm hits your airport and you get grounded for hours and hours, maybe even a day or two. How you initially react depends on your personality. You might become angry, or you might try to be a good sport, smiling and joking with the airline staff who are bearing the brunt of other people's bad tempers. You might start to feel anxious about your home or family, about appointments you've made that now have to be canceled. In the crowd of stranded travelers around you, you will probably witness all these reactions and more. After a few hours, though, a common reaction will start to be obvious. People will become listless, dejected, expressionless, staring emptily at the TV monitors or the crowd. They are depressed, mentally and physically. No scientist has yet gone through an airport crowd seeking volunteers to let their spinal fluid be sampled, but if one did, the scientifically proven finding would likely be low serotonin.

For stranded travelers in an airport, becoming temporarily shut down by depression is arguably a well-adapted response to their frustrating situation. Despite the contemporary tendency to label low mood as an illness that needs to be fixed by therapy or medication, depression can be the best response to a bad situation: "putting your head down and staying out of trouble" versus "beating your head against the wall." A lowering of mood and energy over a series of cold, overcast days may be inconvenient and unnecessary for life in our climate-controlled, artificially lighted environments, but it is a *natural* rather than a *pathological* response. Depression only becomes an illness when the depressed response is chronic, disabling, and out of proportion to one's actual problems and stresses.

A Little Down, or Downright Depressed?

Moods exist on a smooth, flowing continuum—no one behavior or feeling serves to categorize or diagnose a person as truly depressed. Let's take two examples of the almost infinite variety of human mood and behavior.

Nancy's roommates are really worried about her. Since she broke up with her boyfriend a month ago, she cries constantly, refuses to eat, and barely budges out of bed. Her facial expression is flat, wooden, almost zombie-like, and she has lost ten pounds that she didn't need to lose. She keeps saying that she feels worthless, unlovable, and that life isn't worth living. The strange thing about it is, previous to the breakup she never seemed to care that much about her boyfriend.

George has good health, a good job, and a good marriage, but he just doesn't seem to enjoy life as much as he could. He is a little slow to smile and slow to laugh. His personal successes never seem to bring him up, but his mistakes and setbacks really bring him down. He's usually pleasant to be with, but he has good days and bad days. On the bad days, he has a lot of trouble getting up in the morning, finds it hard to concentrate at work, and definitely needs a nightcap to unwind. All the same, he will wake up way too early, full of vague worries. He sometimes masks his what-if worrying by getting irritable with his wife and coworkers.

We don't need to call in a panel of experts to diagnose these two cases. Nancy is truly depressed, and in urgent need of treatment before she hurts herself through malnutrition or more drastic self-harm. George? Well, we all know George. He is our colleague, friend, neighbor, family member, or maybe ourself. George is certainly not sick, but could he be "more well"?

We are accustomed to thinking of people like Nancy as mentally ill and of people like George as "just like that." In fact, these judgments are unfair to both of them, and they have more in common than first appears. George's and Nancy's negative moods and behaviors both involve serotonin system deficiencies, in one case mild, in the other severe.

Over the last twenty years, large numbers of people with mild mood problems similar to George's have tried Prozac, Zoloft, Paxil, or another of the newer antidepressants. Allowing for the fact that successes get more publicity than flops, many people do report mood-elevating results. Behavior that seems to be basic to an individual's character can suddenly change. Shy, withdrawn, cautious persons become bolder, more social, and more outgoing. People whose egos and self-esteem bruise easily, who tend to deflate with each little setback or slight, suddenly become confident, even overconfident, and much more assertive. Wimp becomes hero, wallflower becomes belle of the ball, and the pumpkin turns into a coach.

Is this a recreational use of a drug? Is it similar to the craze and the claims once made for Valium? Some critics have said so. Compared to previous classes of pep and happy pills, the SSRI antidepressants are non-addictive (although they can produce a nasty withdrawal syndrome, as discussed later in the chapter). There is no evidence to say that George should not take an antidepressant, that it will harm his health in any permanent or significant way. Whether George *needs* to take Zoloft, Paxil, or Prozac is a separate question. For people with mild mood problems, the increased physical activity and other lifestyle changes recommended in part three of this book can produce the same mood-elevating effects, without the insomnia, nausea, constipation, sexual problems, withdrawal issues, and other side effects of antidepressants.

Mood Swings and Cycles

While some people are always a little low-key, a little subdued, others bounce up and down the mood spectrum from blue to bubbly, or go back and forth between painfully low and a tolerably neutral mood. People with up-and-down moods may feel like they are strapped into the seat of a roller coaster. Depending on the mood extremes, they may find that they are buoyant and self-assured while they are up, but fatigued and self-doubting when their mood shifts back to low. They may be highly productive during the upswings, or so overexcited that they can barely function. These back-and-forth swings can take place over the course of days, or even within hours. There may be daily, monthly, and seasonal patterns to the swings. If you have mood swings, keeping a Food-Mood-Activity Journal, as explained in chapter 12, will help you to detect any patterns and determine whether your mood swings correlate with your eating patterns and daily habits. Careful attention to how foods, alcohol, and certain activities affect your moods may help you avoid painful lows or uncomfortably over-charged highs.

'Tis the Season to Be SAD

Seasonal affective disorder (SAD) was first recognized and studied by Dr. Norman Rosenthal and his colleagues at the National Institute of Mental Health. In a series of studies published in the 1980s, he identified the symptoms, the causes, and the most effective treatment for this very common problem.

The symptoms will sound very familiar. Beginning in the late fall and continuing through most of the winter, affected individuals will notice a drop in their mood; they will tend to overeat and gain weight; they will feel listless and lethargic; and they will sleep much more than their norm. Come spring, their symptoms will go away, although the weight gained may not.

According to surveys, about half of all people in the northern United States feel worse in the winter, and an estimated one in four Americans has at least mild SAD. A few have other seasonal patterns, such as summer heat intolerance, which is more common in the southern states. Dr. Norman Rosenthal and his colleagues devised a survey to identify people with SAD. The abridged version of it that follows can help you assess your own symptoms. Try to think back over several years of living in the same geographical region, not just the most recent year.

TO WHAT EXTENT DO THE FOLLOWING CHANGE WITH THE SEASONS?

	no change 0	slight change 1	moderate change 2	marked change 3	extremely marked 4
Length of sleep	☐	☐	☐	☐	☐
Social activity	☐	☐	☐	☐	☐
Mood (overall feeling of well-being)	☐	☐	☐	☐	☐
Weight	☐	☐	☐	☐	☐
Appetite	☐	☐	☐	☐	☐
Energy level	☐	☐	☐	☐	☐

Add together your scores for all six items for a total score: _____.
The average person's score falls between 4 and 7 points. A score of 8 to
10 points suggests the milder condition that Dr. Rosenthal calls winter
blues. A score of 11 or higher points indicates a greater likelihood of
SAD. In studies and surveys, people with SAD report sleeping an average of 2.5 hours more in the winter than the summer. People with
milder winter blues sleep about 1.7 hours longer. The average person in
the northeast United States sleeps about 45 minutes longer during the
winter.

If you have winter blues, you may think that you become sad or irritable simply because you hate winter or hate the cold, and you might
explain your increased hunger or extra time in bed as your body's attempts to keep warm. Logical as these explanations may seem, some very
careful studies have shown that the crucial factor is reduced exposure to
bright light.

Light striking the eyes does more than allow us to see. It has a
hormone-like effect on our brain chemistry, as explained in chapter 3.
The best treatment for SAD is increased exposure to bright light,

preferably in the morning. Exercising outdoors when the weather permits, running errands on foot, and working near a window are good, healthy, mood-lifting approaches. Even an overcast winter day is much brighter than a well-lit office. If you have SAD symptoms, don't wear sunglasses in the fall and winter, unless the glare really does bother you.

Why do we get SAD? Perhaps some degree of SAD-ness served as a useful adaptation to living in colder climates, helping early humans deal with their reduced level of activity during the long nights. In a 2001 study (published in *Archives of General Psychiatry*), researchers from the National Institute of Mental Health found that people with SAD have kept that adaptation (which we share with animals), while the rest of us have lost it. Under uniform dim light conditions, patients with SAD had a longer nighttime period of melatonin secretion in winter than in summer, a difference not seen in a matched group of healthy non-SAD volunteers. Since we spend most of our days and evenings under artificial lighting that is roughly five hundred times brighter than the very dim lights used in this experiment, it is not quite clear how this difference in melatonin production plays out under normal living conditions, but it is an important clue to a real biological difference underlying SAD.

The symptoms of SAD are decidedly worsened by the fact that modern humans spend most of their days and evenings under artificial light, with very limited exposure to daylight. The brain's clock (a function of the hypothalamus) is powerfully affected by dusk and dawn, which act as a pair of clock timers to turn melatonin production on and off. According to the phase-shift theory of winter depression proposed by researcher Alfred Lewy, one of the clock timers, usually the dawn melatonin-off switch, is still set to the summer schedule. These SAD people do not have sufficient daylight exposure, especially in the early morning, to get their body's sleep-wake, melatonin-serotonin cycle properly cued to the change of season.

Some seasonal changes affect us all. During the winter, serotonin levels drop in the hypothalamus, the part of the brain regulating sleep and appetite, even for individuals who do not have symptoms of SAD. Reduced serotonin levels in the hypothalamus have shown a strong link to increased appetite and overeating in both humans and animals. Maybe second helpings of Thanksgiving stuffing and all the Christmas partying have been unfairly blamed for the all-too-common experience of a winter weight gain.

People with SAD do overeat as part of the syndrome, but they don't tend to eat more of every food group. Instead, they report a sometimes overwhelming craving for carbohydrates—either sweet or starchy ones. During the SAD season, they will tend to fill up on bread, pasta, and potatoes at meals, and perhaps seek out cupcakes or other sweet snacks between meals. Not only are these carbohydrate foods more tempting, their consumption is usually rewarded with an energy boost and better spirits for the next hour or half hour. Of course, the weight gain that results from increased eating and snacking can have a much more lasting negative impact on body image and self-esteem.

If you are a wintertime binge eater, consider this idea before you beat up on yourself for your lack of will power. A number of researchers now believe this craving for carbohydrates is a form of self-medication. A properly timed carbohydrate meal *will* raise levels of brain tryptophan, from which serotonin is formed. If you crave carbohydrates during the winter, or year round, to give yourself an energy and mood boost, chapters 8 and 9 will give you guidance in choosing foods that will increase your energy but not your weight.

If your SAD symptoms are mild to moderate, the dietary and other lifestyle changes described in part three can be effective in minimizing the negative impact of winter on your mood, eating, and sleep patterns. The prevention and treatment solution may be as simple as getting outside in the early morning for a half hour or so. For more severe symptoms, the recommended treatment is light therapy, usually delivered by a small tabletop light box or panel. Before investing in this fairly expensive equipment, you should certainly consult a doctor to be sure your symptoms are SAD. Light-box therapy is not effective for non-SAD depression and other mood and eating disorders. Some health insurance policies will cover costs of the equipment if you do have a medical diagnosis. If you have migraine or other chronic headaches, you may want to rent a unit first to be sure the bright light will not bring on further attacks.

Compare the lux as well as the prices if you are shopping around for one of these units. (The *lux* is a rather arbitrary unit for measuring light intensity.) Ordinary indoor lighting ranges from 100 to 1,000 lux. The standard prescription for bright light therapy, either for SAD or delayed sleep phase insomnia, is 5,000 lux daily in the early morning. A light therapy box that delivers 10,000 lux of light is usually effective in resetting the circadian clock with a half hour of daily use, while a light panel that delivers 2,500 lux would need to be used for two hours daily. Most of the better units are portable, so you can take one to work with you for use as a desk light. You don't have to stare into the light in order to get its benefits, and you can read or work while you are getting your daily dose of light, so long as you stay close to the unit. For SAD sufferers, light therapy appears to act as a natural energizing antidepressant, either by increasing serotonin levels, decreasing norepinephrine levels, resetting the internal day-night clock, or some complex combination of effects. As another alternative, the antidepressant Welbutrin XL (extended release) recently obtained FDA approval as a treatment for SAD. There is no evidence, however, that Welbutrin or any of the other antidepressants are more effective than light therapy.

Serotonin in PMS

There are over 150 reported symptoms of premenstrual syndrome, and the great majority of women experience at least mild PMS in the days directly before their period. Among the most common premenstrual changes are:

- Mood, energy, and attention: irritability, nervousness, agitation, difficulty concentrating, fatigue, depression, mood swings, tension
- Sleep: insomnia

- Gastrointestinal symptoms: bloating, constipation, nausea, vomiting
- Behavior and appetite: bingeing, anorexia, cravings, lack of impulse control, poor performance at work or school, avoiding social activities
- Water retention (edema): temporary weight gain, breast tenderness, swelling
- Nervous system and blood vessels: headache, dizziness, cold sweats, numbness or changed sensation in extremities, easy bruising, heart pounding
- Worsening of chronic problems: acne and other skin problems, allergies, respiratory complaints, visual disturbances, conjunctivitis (pinkeye)

A few of the most common physical symptoms, such as temporary weight gain and swelling, result from the direct effects of the hormones estrogen and progesterone on water retention. The most troubling features of PMS, of course, are the mood, food craving, and pain symptoms, which can range from barely noticeable to quite disabling. PMS symptoms can come and go within a few hours, or persist for ten days or longer—a full third of the monthly cycle for women with prolonged PMS. PMS that is dominated by severe mood symptoms has been labeled premenstrual dysphoric disorder (PMDD). It is believed, for obvious reasons, that fluctuations in estrogen and progesterone levels must somehow account for all these symptoms, but the mechanisms are not really known. These hormones readily pass into the brain, where they interact with neurotransmitter systems. Their fluctuations late in the cycle launch a series of chemical changes that include changes in the serotonin system.

The mood, sleep, pain, and food-craving symptoms of PMS all point strongly to the involvement of serotonin. In animals and in laboratory experiments, levels of estrogen, progesterone, and other hormones have been shown to influence serotonin availability to a marked degree, with different effects apparent in different parts of the brain. Estrogen has very complex effects on the serotonin system, but the overall trend is clear:

high estrogen, high serotonin; low estrogen, low serotonin. The symptoms of PMS occur at the low estrogen point of a woman's monthly hormonal fluctuations. Clinical studies have found fluctuations in serotonin activity throughout the menstrual cycle that show a close correlation to mood changes. A 1989 study in the *American Journal of Clinical Nutrition* reported that the ways the female body breaks down and uses tryptophan is different at different stages in the menstrual cycle—a possible reason for the mood and food symptoms experienced in PMS.

Following the controversial redefinition of severe PMS as a psychiatric illness, the pharmaceutical companies responded to this new market opportunity by launching clinical trials of their antidepressants for women diagnosed with PMDD. Eli Lilly was the first to score, gaining FDA approval to market Prozac for PMDD in 2000 under the new brand name of Sarafem (which presumably sounds more feminine). Paxil and Zoloft have also been approved for this new indication. PMDD is defined as severe premenstrual distress (irritability, anger, anxiety, depression) and is estimated to affect only 3 to 8 percent of women in their reproductive years, compared to 75 to 80 percent for plain old PMS. Yet, because of diagnosis creep, the prescriptions may be handed out much more liberally than those numbers suggest.

Certainly, women who do have severe mood problems with their premenstrual symptoms should consider trying antidepressants, but the efficacy rates in the clinical trials have been fairly low, in the range of 35 to 50 percent. As for other options, oral contraceptives and other hormonal treatments sometimes help and sometimes make symptoms worse. Although medical treatments are limited, better nutrition (less animal fat, more fiber), vitamin supplementation (B-complex vitamins), and exercise have been reported successful in improving symptoms, and so has behavioral training in reducing stress and tension. Dietary and lifestyle modifications are covered in detail in part three of this book.

Although PMS is a hormonal rather than a psychological condition, your mood and mind-set as your period approaches undoubtedly play a role in reducing or heightening your symptoms. If you dread the onset of PMS and feel helpless, your depression, irritability, and tearfulness will likely be much worse. A simple "take control" step such as getting more exercise in the pre-PMS days can have a physiological *and* psychological impact on how you feel as your monthly period approaches.

Depression in Women: Is It Estrogen or Environment?

As discussed in chapter 2, women have two times the risk of major depression and three times the risk of borderline depression (called dysthymia) that men do. The negative moods of PMS and PMDD are obviously 100 percent a problem of women in their childbearing years. Women seem to be much more subject to fluctuations in serotonin activity than men, due largely to the effects of estrogen. The points in the life cycle when estrogen is lowest—the premenstrual days, the weeks after childbirth (baby blues, or postpartum depression), and menopause—are the times when women are at increased risk of episodes of emotional ups and downs or outright depression. Estrogen replacement therapy has been shown to improve mood for menopausal women troubled by depressed, tearful, or anxious moods. The effects of testosterone on serotonin activity have received less attention. The few animal studies that have been done suggest that testosterone, unlike estrogen, may exert a stabilizing influence on the serotonin system, lessening the effects of diet, environment, and drugs on serotonin activity.

But "It's all because of estrogen" is a non-answer, equivalent to saying, "Women are just like that." At some point in human history, or in our animal past, there likely was a survival advantage to the depressed response that was more powerful for females than males. Today, when most of us live in towns and cities ranging in population from a few thousand to several million, depression is often linked to being isolated and alone. We lose sight of the fact that our ancestors lived in tiny villages or tribal groups where everyone knew everyone else, no one was ever alone, and depression was linked to being unpopular or low in social status. Traditional societies functioned more like unsupervised children in the schoolyard—jostling for rank, bullying the weak, ostracizing the unpopular.

In this context, depressed behavior (submissiveness) is thought to have evolved as a way of signaling defeat, to avoid further conflict with the dominant members of one's group, a strategy of damage control. It is a behavior pattern that can be observed in many social species. Female monkeys, who also have monthly menstrual cycles, have been studied as a model for how estrogen affects brain and behavior. Studies involving small colonies of female monkeys have shown that bullied, subordinate females exhibit depressed behavior and have reduced serotonin functioning, particularly under low-estrogen conditions.

Of course, neither monkeys nor humans live in all-female societies. Under normal conditions, some females are dominant over other females, some males are dominant over other males, but the males generally dominate the females. An old American folk ballad, "The Wagoner's Lad," nicely summarizes the subordinate status of women in the traditional world:

> Oh hard is the fortune of all womankind,
> She's always controlled, she's always confined.
> Controlled by her parents until she's a wife,
> Then slave to her husband for the rest of her life.

If depression functions as a survival mechanism that keeps you from starting fights you can't win, then it makes sense that females would have a greater likelihood of responding to stress and struggle with depression.

Serotonin and Mood in Schizophrenia

Schizophrenia is a surprisingly common disease, afflicting one percent of the population. It is now known to be a disease, like diabetes or muscular dystrophy. The many theories that claimed bad parenting was its cause have been abandoned since we have learned more about the brain chemical imbalances that occur with this disease. It tends to be inherited, and it most often strikes in the late teens or early twenties, frequently in response to the stress of leaving home for college or beginning employment. The most striking symptoms are delusional ideas and hallucinations, such as hearing voices that say disturbing or frightening things. People with schizophrenia also tend to lose their normal responsiveness and expressiveness, seeming flat, withdrawn, and without interest in anything or anybody. At the same time, they can have severe impulse control problems. They may become antisocial and aggressive, either uncooperative or actually violent, a danger to themselves and others. Suicide attempts are common, often in response to the voices that only the sufferer can hear, voices that may tell them that they are bad, worthless people, or that command them to jump from a window or swallow poison.

The main chemical culprit in schizophrenia appears to be the neurotransmitter dopamine, which is overly active in certain parts of the brain of schizophrenic persons. The mood and impulse symptoms of schizophrenia are thought to be related to abnormalities in the serotonin system. Medical treatment of schizophrenia relies on a class of medications called atypical antipsychotics, which includes Clozaril (clozapine), Risperdal (risperidone), Zyprexa (olanzapine), Seroquel (quetiapine) among others. These drugs act on both the dopamine and serotonin systems and are effective in improving both groups of symptoms—the delusions and hallucinations, and the mood and impulse (flat, depressed, withdrawn, aggressive, suicidal) symptoms. In many cases these medications have allowed people to live normal or near-normal lives. These drugs treat the disease without reversing the underlying neurotransmitter abnormalities, so they must be taken for life to avoid a relapse. Recent preliminary studies have also suggested potential benefits from combining a serotonin-active antinausea drug, such as Navoban (tropisetron) or Zofran (ondansetron) with standard antipsychotic medications.

Serotonin and Parkinson's Disease

Parkinson's disease is another common disease linked to neurotransmitter imbalances. The main symptoms of Parkinson's disease are tremor, muscular stiffness or rigidity, and a slowness in movement accompanied by difficulty in beginning movement that is called bradykinesia. Trembling in an arm or hand while resting or under stress is often the first symptom. As it progresses over years, Parkinson's sufferers have to consciously relearn how to make simple movements, such as walking or sitting down, that are so natural and unconscious in normal health. It is most often a disease beginning later in life, between ages fifty and eighty. It is neither hereditary nor contagious, and the triggering cause is not understood. (A look-alike condition called parkinsonism, or Parkinson's syndrome, can be traced to specific injuries, diseases, and drugs.) The symptoms of Parkinson's disease are known to result from neurotransmitter imbalances, following the loss of nerve cells that produce dopamine. This imbalance can be partially remedied through drug treatment. Over time, however, drugs becomes less and less effective in controlling the symptoms.

People with Parkinson's often suffer from severe depression. You might say, "Who wouldn't, with such a terrible disease," but sometimes depression and anxiety are among the first symptoms, appearing before the disease has been diagnosed. Studies reveal that persons with Parkinson's are more prone to depression than other people with progressive and disabling diseases. This finding suggests that changes in the balance of dopamine and serotonin may be responsible for the depression. Antidepressants can not only relieve the depression but also have mild benefits in improving the primary movement symptoms.

Serotonin and Alzheimer's Disease

Over 4.5 million Americans have Alzheimer's disease, yet medical researchers do not yet know what causes it. A genetic abnormality has been identified in some cases, but most researchers believe environmental factors, such as viruses or contaminants, must have an important role. The symptoms result from the loss of cells in several key areas of the brain and reduced availability of the neurotransmitter acetylcholine, which is important to memory. There are several puzzling abnormalities in the brain that could be either a cause or a result of the disease's progression, including abnormal deposits, or plaques, and strange growths called tangles. Recently, a sophisticated PET brain imaging study of Alzheimer's patients discovered a profound loss of a specific serotonin receptor (5-HT$_{1A}$) in the hippocampus (which is the brain region crucial to memory). This decline in receptor density may simply be a marker for the degeneration of the brain cells themselves, but it is likely to be linked with disease symptoms such as agitation and anxiety.

The most striking change in Alzheimer's is of course the loss of memory functioning. Sufferers will lose both the ability to learn new information and the ability to recall most past learning. These changes are progressive, usually over several years. Alzheimer's victims also can have changes in mood and behavior that are even more distressing to their families than the loss of mental functioning. They can become severely anxious and depressed, or they may become aggressive and uncooperative, biting and scratching their caregivers as they attempt to bathe or dress them. In later stages of the disease there may be a complete loss of sexual inhibition and attempts to have sex with anyone within reach. Often families who are able to cope with the mental deterioration find they have to put their parent or spouse into a nursing home because of the behavior changes.

It is certainly the case that people with Alzheimer's disease may be consciously depressed and anxious early in the course of the disease, as they experience the gradual loss of their ability to function and to take care of themselves. In the later stages, the confusion felt by patients who can no longer understand what is going on around them might explain the anxiety, agitation, and aggressiveness of their responses. While these psychological explanations make sense, it is also very likely that the serotonin system is involved. In postmortem examinations, severe abnormalities in the serotonin system can be found in the brain. Serotonin is known to have a role in memory, as well as in mood, aggression, and impulse control.

Prozac and other SSRI antidepressants have been effective in controlling the mood and behavior changes of many Alzheimer's patients, sometimes making it possible to care for them at home longer or in a less restricted nursing home setting. This is a significant benefit, particularly since the treatments available for the loss of memory and mental functioning have only modest efficacy.

All About Antidepressants

As explained in chapter 2, most (but not all) antidepressants act in some way to increase the availability of serotonin in the brain or the activity of the serotonin system. Despite their name, antidepressants are prescribed for much more than depression. They have been used to treat a wide range of eating, mood, pain, and impulse or addiction problems—basically any condition in which serotonin is known to have a role.

Many familiar drugs were discovered serendipitously by chemists screening hundreds and thousands of compounds for possible beneficial effects. As the first of the SSRI antidepressants (others in this class are Zoloft, Celexa, Lexapro, and Paxil), Prozac was celebrated as an early triumph of the modern era of "designer" or "targeted" drugs. The SSRIs ("selective serotonin reuptake inhibitors") were designed specifically to increase serotonin availability in the brain by blocking the action of the serotonin transporter (also called SERT), which regulates the amount of serotonin available.

However, more recent research, as summarized in chapter 2, has found that people who have a genetic variant of SERT that is a less efficient serotonin transporter have a greater risk of depression, so it is now hard to understand why blocking SERT would be therapeutic for these patients. Moreover, these antidepressants have an immediate effect on increasing brain serotonin levels, but an unexplained time lag of two to four weeks in actually relieving the symptoms of depression. The prescribing information for these drugs now includes some acknowledgment of uncertainty: "The precise action of SSRIs is not fully understood."

Sometimes a person who gets nothing but side effects from one antidepressant has good results with another. No one can really predict or explain why antidepressants work or don't work in any given situation. Tofranil, an older drug that acted on the norepinephrine system with very little direct effect on serotonin, was an effective antidepressant. Some of the newer antidepressants target both the serotonin and norepinephrine systems (for example, Cymbalta and Effexor). Apparently, the brain is more like a Rube Goldberg machine (prone to complex, unpredictable chain reactions) than a recipe for cookies. Drugs acting on serotonin or norepinephrine availability will trigger a series of adjustments in serotonin functioning as well as in other neurotransmitter systems. One or more of these changes act to relieve depression.

Prozac and the other SSRI antidepressants have never been shown to be more effective than older classes of antidepressants, the monoamine oxidase inhibitors (MAOIs) and the tricyclic antidepressants. As the first of the SSRI antidepressants, Prozac's main contribution—the one that propelled it to stardom—was fewer and more acceptable side effects. The tricyclic antidepressants (such as Norpramin, Elavil, and Vivactil) produce a set of side effects called anticholinergic that are similar to the side effects of over-the-counter antihistamines taken for colds and allergies. Dry mouth is a common complaint while taking one of these antidepressants, and this side effect often doesn't improve much over time. Weight gain, drowsiness, and blurred vision are other unpopular side effects. Anticholinergic side effects can also include memory problems—resulting from the drug's interference with the activity of acetylcholine. Declines in short-term memory are sometimes noticeable in elderly persons taking tricyclic antidepressants, but usually not in younger ones. Because of the universally disliked side effects, people tended to stop their medication or drop out of treatment, and physicians didn't prescribe the drugs unless someone had true depression, not just moodiness or blues. The tricyclic antidepressants are still preferred to the SSRI antidepressants for some serotonin-related conditions, including chronic pain.

The MAOIs (only Parnate is still on the market) are very effective in relieving depression and also in treating migraine. However, they have been even less prescribed because of a potentially very dangerous food-drug interaction. Anyone taking an MAOI must avoid all foods with high levels of the amino acid tyramine, found in aged, fermented, and smoked foods, including sour cream and yogurt, pickled herring, red wine and beer, and cheese. Consuming large quantities of tyramine while taking an MAOI can drastically raise blood pressure to dangerous, life-threatening levels. Antihistamines, such as cold and allergy remedies, must also be avoided. The MAOIs are particularly risky for serotonin syndrome (as discussed in chapter 2).

In contrast, the newer antidepressants caused fewer and less frequent side effects and are not nearly as dangerous in overdose. Some people have nausea and insomnia for the first weeks of treatment, and some degree of constipation is also common and may persist throughout treatment. Sexual problems also occur, primarily delayed ejaculation or orgasm, although some of the pharmaceutical companies have spun this into a benefit by positioning their drug as a treatment for premature ejaculation. Headaches can be a problem, even though these drugs sometimes successfully treat chronic headache.

In the years immediately after its introduction in 1987, Prozac became a pharmaceutical bestseller, the first socially acceptable antidepressant. People who would not have considered taking one of the older antidepressants, or wouldn't have talked about it if they did, raved about how Prozac had transformed their lives. Because of their perceived safety and acceptability, physicians felt more comfortable with prescribing the

SSRI antidepressants, and more willing to do so in situations where some-one wasn't clearly or severely in need of drug treatment for depression. The FDA-approved indications for these drugs have expanded steadily over the last two decades. Fluoxetine (the generic name for Prozac and Sarafem) is now approved as a treatment for not just depression but also panic disorder, obsessive-compulsive disorder, bulimia, and premenstrual dysphoric disorder (PMS with mood symptoms). Its off-label uses (unap-proved by the FDA) include alcoholism, anorexia nervosa, anxiety, autism, borderline personality disorder, fibromyalgia, hot flashes, menopause, obesity, and premature ejaculation. Zoloft and Paxil are both approved for depression, anxiety, obsessive-compulsive disorder, panic disorder, post-traumatic stress disorder, premenstrual dysphoric disorder, and "so-cial anxiety disorder" (what used to be called being painfully shy). De-spite the millions of prescriptions written for these drugs over the past twenty years, there is still much unresolved controversy over both their efficacy and their safety.

The Unsuspected Power of a Placebo

A placebo is a look-alike dummy medication that is used in clinical drug comparison studies. Before a new drug is approved for use by the FDA, it must be proven more effective than either an already approved drug or a placebo in a double-blind study (meaning that neither the doctors nor the patients know who is getting what kind of pill). Most of the FDA-approved antidepressants were tested against a placebo. You might think that is an easy standard to meet—the drug simply has to be better than nothing! The problem is that placebos are surprisingly effective—often nearly as effective as the active medication.

In a 2003 study appearing in the journal *Neuropsychopharmacology,* a team of researchers used the Freedom of Information Act to obtain access to data from double-blind trials reported to the FDA in support of nine antidepressants that were eventually approved by the FDA. The researchers' objective was to look at the effect of study design on outcome. They found that the response rates to the antidepressants in these studies ranged from 28 to 61 percent. In the placebo groups, the response rates ranged from 10 to 42 percent. *The antidepressant was statistically better than the placebo in only 58 percent of the studies, yet all nine antidepressants were ultimately approved as effective by the FDA.*

When you consider that these trials were funded by the drug companies, who hired the investigators and approved the study design and in many cases did the data analysis, the evidence they were able to muster to show their products' efficacy is far from impressive. A response rate of 55 percent for Effexor sounds respectable, until you learn that the placebo response in the same trial was 39 percent. Researchers consider that the true response rate is revealed by subtracting the placebo response from the drug response—making it 16 percent in this instance. Antidepressants do work, but only for some people, some of the time. Others get better on their own (although they may credit the antidepressant with the improvement), or keep trying one medication after another.

For approval of a new antidepressant, the FDA's standard is a minimum of two placebo-controlled studies showing a statistically significant advantage for the drug, but the number of unsuccessful or negative studies does not count against the application for approval. Additional problems with these studies include the fact that patients often figure out that they are getting a placebo when they have no side effects, and placebo responders have been known to relapse if they find out the treatment is a sham. Also, the symptom assessment questionnaire used to measure treatment success in these trials is very general. It includes questions about anxiety and sleep, so that a drug that had mostly sedative effects could be scored as an effective antidepressant. Research is ongoing to try to develop better clinical trial designs to truly demonstrate what is medication effect versus placebo effect.

In the past, doctors would sometimes prescribe "sugar pills" for patients who kept complaining about vague symptoms. If the patient got better on the placebo, that was taken as proof that he or she had not really been sick, or perhaps that the illness improved on its own. Today there is a greater realization that placebo treatment can actually relieve symptoms, particularly in pain and mood disorders, perhaps by stimulating the body's natural painkillers, or by other more mysterious self-healing processes. These improvements can be temporary or long-lasting. This unexplained improvement with a dummy treatment, which occurs with many different diseases and disorders, is called the placebo effect.

It is thought that every treatment, real or fake, has a placebo effect that is proportionate to the recipient's faith and hope in its efficacy. Wise healers in every tradition, Eastern, Western, and alternative therapies, draw upon the healing power of the placebo effect when the empathy and interest they communicate raises the patient's confidence in the healer and hope for a cure. The peace of mind we get from confiding a problem to a trusted friend might also be a manifestation of the placebo effect, in this instance, of the healing influence of sympathy and positive encouragement.

The "healing power of hope" sounds phony and clichéd. But something real does takes place in the brain with a placebo effect. A brain activity study reported in 2002 in the *American Journal of Psychiatry* found that placebo responders had distinct changes in brain activity patterns in the prefrontal cortex (which has a key role in interpreting experience) that were not present in nonresponders to either placebo or antidepressant medication. Interestingly, a distinct set of brain activity changes were seen in the patients who responded to drug treatment. Either placebo or antidepressant medication can relieve the symptoms of depression, but by different mechanisms. In this study, 52 percent of patients improved on antidepressant therapy and 38 percent achieved a comparable improvement on placebo treatment.

The placebo response seems to be particularly powerful in mild to moderate depression. In some studies, in fact, the placebo group improved more than those getting the antidepressant! Mood disorders tend to cycle up and down, from better to worse, from worse to better. If people seek help (or medication) when they are at their lowest point, then they may be headed for an upswing regardless of treatment. The very act of seeking treatment—being hopeful and active rather than helpless and passive—is itself a temporary antidepressant.

Antidepressants may be life changing, even life saving, for people who truly need them. But if your mood problems are not severe, is taking a pill a better approach to life's problems than taking action? As Joanna Moncrieff, a critic of the pharmaceutical industry's claims for antidepressants, has observed, "The prescription of medication for depression conveys the powerful message that we are passive victims of our biology." And then there's the issue of side effects.

The Dark Side of Antidepressants

Moncrieff is among the researchers who have analyzed the pharmaceutical industry–sponsored trials and have questioned whether antidepressants have a truly meaningful benefit for depression. This is a minority view, although a legitimate one; most physicians and researchers believe antidepressants are effective, although not nearly so effective as their ad campaigns claim. Certainly, no one has ever suggested that antidepressants do *nothing*: They undoubtedly have real, though poorly understood, effects on the brain. These effects appear to have positive, activating consequences for many individuals with depression, lifting them out of passivity and despondency and allowing them to get on with their lives. Some people will get agitated or hyperactive in response to the change to their brain chemistry. A lower dosage or a different drug will usually remedy the problem. For a small number—for still unknown reasons—the activating effects of these drugs lead to acts of self-mutilation or impulsive suicide attempts.

Beginning in 1990, there were a number of reports that patients taking SSRI antidepressants had become suicidal. The researchers who looked closely at these early cases (mostly involving fluoxetine, or Prozac) came to the conclusion that the drug had raised these patients' energy level without giving them needed impulse control. Apparently, some people who are severely depressed will initially respond to a powerful serotonin-active drug by being able to act on violent or suicidal ideas and impulses that had been hidden beneath their extreme lack of energy and motivation.

As additional SSRI antidepressants were developed and approved by the FDA, the pharmaceutical companies successfully sought to expand their market by studies designed to establish their drugs' effectiveness for other mood disorders (such as anxiety and obsessive-compulsive disorder) and for other patient populations (children and adolescents). But as the number of prescriptions increased, so did the reports of violence, suicide, and other acts of self-harm in patients on these drugs, particularly among adolescents.

An analysis (which appeared in *The Lancet* in 2004) of all the available studies of SSRI antidepressants for childhood depression found that the pharmaceutical companies had routinely suppressed publication of unfavorable data, including suicides and serious side effects. The researchers concluded that the risks outweigh the benefits of these drugs (with the exception of fluoxetine) in treating depression in children and adolescents. Rather belatedly, the FDA has now required that the prescribing information for all the antidepressants include a black box warning of the risk of suicidal behavior in children and adolescents.

Similar analyses have been made of all the available studies to examine whether adult patients also show an increase in suicidal behavior while on SSRI antidepressants. The link is less clear in the older population, but there are enough worrying signs that the FDA is now undertaking a full review of all its data from hundreds of reported trials. Although most of these formal analyses involved only the SSRI antidepressants (Zoloft, Celexa, Lexapro, Paxil, and Prozac), the SNRI antidepressants (Effexor and Cymbalta) are also associated with an increased occurrence of suicidal behavior.

The risks of suicidal or violent behavior seem to be limited to the first few months of treatment or to increases in dosage or other changes in medication. But there is another risk at the *end* of treatment that people on antidepressants need to know about: Abruptly stopping treatment with any antidepressant can bring on a withdrawal syndrome that includes such unpleasant effects as dizziness, gastrointestinal upset, either lethargy or an anxious hyperactivity, low mood, sleep problems, and headache. Slow tapering of doses usually avoids the withdrawal symptoms.

Should You Take an Antidepressant?

Anyone who has severe problems with mood, chronic headache, or controlling their eating and drinking should consult a doctor or an appropriate therapist, period. You need to rule out the possibility that there is a serious underlying medical condition and to learn about the full range of treatments available. If you are opposed to taking antidepressants, there are a number of behavioral approaches that can help. These basically work by identifying and then changing the negative, unhealthy ways your mind and body respond to stress and setbacks. Biofeedback and relaxation techniques help with anxiety and chronic headache; cognitive therapy is effective for both depression and anxiety. There are behavior therapies specifically designed for eating disorders and addiction. You also should not underestimate the healing power of the sympathy and understanding you can get from a knowing professional.

For all the concerns about the safety and true efficacy rates of antidepressants, the fact remains that they have been taken by millions of people with only minor side effects. They are more effective than a placebo, although perhaps not by a large margin. They do relieve symptoms of depression, although their mechanism of action is not known. Until something better comes along (and is stringently tested for safety and efficacy), people with severe mood disorders may be best benefited by a combination of psychotherapy and medication.

How Long Do You Have to Take It?
Six Weeks? Or a Lifetime?

Aspirin either relieves a headache within a few minutes, or it doesn't. Antidepressants are much less predictable. Although laboratory experiments show an immediate effect on the serotonin system receptors, as already noted, in real life and real brains, antidepressants do not begin to work for two weeks to a month after starting treatment. No one has quite explained why there is such a long delay between beginning treatment and seeing improvement. (The current best guess is based on the observation that, in animal studies, these drugs increase the production of new cells in the brain's memory center, the hippocampus, over the course of the first few weeks of treatment.)

There is no established length of treatment. In the past, therapists often used antidepressants only long enough to get a client out of a crisis, then depended upon psychotherapy to achieve long-term changes in behavior and mood. Since the advent of the newer antidepressants, people now routinely stay on medication, if the side effects are tolerable, for six months to several years. There is no consensus among psychiatrists and therapists for when it is time for a client to come off an antidepressant.

People who have had multiple episodes of severe depression or who became psychotic or suicidal while depressed may well require antidepressant therapy indefinitely, perhaps for life. Those who become depressed following a major life stress, such as divorce, unemployment, or death of a loved one, often stay on antidepressants until they have rebuilt their lives in some meaningful and satisfying way. For people with mild-to-moderate mood problems, it's not clear how long they should take antidepressants, since in the past they generally weren't treated with drugs at all.

It is obviously a matter of choice and preference for the individual therapist and client. Even if the side effects have been minimal, most people would like to reach the point where they are able to replace the energy and ego boost they get from an antidepressant with the energy and ego boost of doing it for themselves—getting the training wheels off their lives and becoming drug free.

If you are currently taking an antidepressant for mild-to-moderate mood disorders, following the nutrition and lifestyle guidelines explained in part three of this book may reduce your need for antidepressant treatment and help you keep your mood and motivation high when it is time for you to taper off your medication. If you are undecided or uncomfortable about taking antidepressants, making the nutrition and lifestyle changes suggested in part three, while keeping a Mood-Food-Activity Journal to track your progress, will allow you to see if you can lick your mood problems on your own.

5

Feeling Pain: Migraine, Irritable Bowel Syndrome, Fibromyalgia

Perhaps there are those who have never had problems with depression, anxiety, insomnia, or overeating, but there is no one—almost no one— who has not felt pain. A few rare individuals have a deficient sense of pain in part or all of their bodies—and are enormously handicapped by it. Diabetics often suffer nerve damage that reduces sensation in their hands and feet. They must inspect their feet continually to avoid over-looking a festering sore or infection that might progress and require am-putation. Without the pain sensations that warn us of risk and injury, we would be in constant danger from burns, frostbite, lacerations, and re-peated stress to muscles, joints, and ligaments that would soon cripple us.

Some people feel chronic pain in the absence of a disease or a lasting injury to the body. Migraine and cluster headaches can be so severe that they are incapacitating, yet there is no underlying disease and no abnor-mality in the brain that can be detected on X rays, CT scans, or MRIs. While common tension-type headache is a mild "take two aspirin and it goes away" condition for most people, more than 45 million Americans are thought to have headaches on a regular basis. (The average American misses five and a half days of school or work per year on account of headaches.) Some people have chronic back pain but do not have a ruptured disk or any other abnormality that could explain the pain. Altogether, some 10 to 30 percent of Americans suffer from some sort of chronic pain condition. All told, the personal and economic toll of chronic pain is considerable.

Why Do We Feel Pain?

We feel pain when special receptors on sensory nerves respond to an irritant that can relate to temperature, to trauma or mechanical forces, or to chemical factors, either the body's own pain-triggering chemicals or toxic substances we eat or get on our skin. The nerves supplying the skin and the neighboring tissues have many pain receptors, and so do the nerves of the gut. Pain receptors also occur on nerves supplying the blood vessels of the brain and body. These pain-sensing nerves send signals to the spinal cord and then onward to the brain. Return signals, moving at speeds up to 100 feet per second, cause us to react to escape the pain, if we can.

Suppose you touch a hot stove. Before you can say or even think "Ouch!" you yank your finger off the stove. This reflex doesn't even involve the brain. The sensory nerve signal travels to the spinal cord where it causes another nerve to contract the muscles of the arm involuntarily, saving you from a much worse burn. The initial pain signal travels onward into the lower part of the brain, called the brain stem, and makes its report. Within the brain stem is a pain center that includes part of the serotonin system. This pain center has a significant role in assessing just how bad the pain is, before passing the message on to other centers that continue to process and respond to the pain signals. You do not actually become aware of the pain until the brain has done its complicated job of processing the information supplied by the nerves.

The initial intense, focused pain sensation is usually followed by a dull, aching pain that is much more persistent. Someone who is distracted or preoccupied at the moment of injury may feel very little of that pain until some time later. On the other hand, someone who is always in fear of the next headache attack, abdominal cramp, or joint twinge will be keenly aware of the first dull throbs of returning pain.

Adding Insult to Injury—Inflammation

When the brain has processed the pain information, a return message is sent to the nerves supplying the injury. This is the point at which you will actually become aware of some painful sensation, such as burning, throbbing, lacerating, searing, or just plain aching. This is also the point at which the body itself attempts to combat the injury and do damage control by launching the inflammatory response.

Everyone has had a cut, burn, sprain, or other injury that gets red, swollen, and much more tender and painful in the hours after the injury took place. This is not part of the injury but part of the healing process. Blood supply to the area increases (causing the warmness and reddening), and the blood vessels in the area begin to leak fluids (resulting in swelling) into the wounded tissue. The fluids contain white blood cells that scout for trouble in the injured tissue and other substances, such as histamine and serotonin, that also take part in the response to injury. Serotonin causes the release and activation of other substances that help to wall off the injury and combat any possible infection. The substances released include prostaglandins, bradykinin, and substance P—all of which can increase the sense of pain and irritation in the damaged tissue. Basically, this response helps to quarantine the injured tissue and its fluids from the rest of the body—a defensive move in case bacteria attack the damaged or weakened cells.

The inflammatory response is essential for protecting the body from bacteria and from toxic substances that enter the body through a wound. However, as everyone with a sprained ankle or tennis elbow well knows, the inflammation can be vastly more painful, more incapacitating, and longer lasting than the injury itself. Usually, though, the inflammatory response is a self-contained and time-limited process. Other chemicals, such as the endorphins, are also released both within the brain and at the site of injury to moderate the message of the pain-inducing chemicals. Even if the inflammation is worse than the injury itself, both will heal, and the pain gradually goes away.

In chronic pain, this process becomes a vicious cycle in which the inflammation perpetuates the pain, and vice versa. Chronic pain can result from chronic diseases, or it can occur because of inherited biochemical abnormalities, such as a relative deficiency of the pain-suppressing neurotransmitters, serotonin, and the endorphins. Sometimes an injury or disease initiates changes in the nerves and muscles that will amplify and prolong the pain. This can occur with injuries to the back or to the jaw (the temporal mandibular joint, or TMJ). The muscles continue to be sore, and specific "trigger points" are tender and painful. The sufferer responds by avoiding use of the muscles, which become further weakened and prone to reinjury.

Serotonin and Pain

Both the pain center in the brain stem and a second pain-processing center, in an area called the thalamus, are richly supplied with serotonin system nerve cells. These cells can send signals back down the spinal cord that interfere with or suppress the pain messages being forwarded from the nerves in the injured area. Within the brain, serotonin interacts with other pain and sensory centers and has the ability to inhibit pain response or pain awareness. Although it has many other functions, serotonin is classified by some researchers as one of the endorphins, the body's natural opium- or morphine-like pain modulators.

A great deal of evidence exists to link migraine and irritable bowel syndrome (IBS) with serotonin abnormalities. For other chronic pain conditions, such as back pain and arthritis, serotonin system deficiencies are not thought to be the source of the problem. Increasing serotonin availability has been shown to decrease pain for a wide variety of persistent or recurrent pain problems. Although the inflammation of arthritis or joint disease may cause the pain, the pain may be made much worse if serotonin availability is low. Antidepressants have been used successfully to reduce pain in chronic headache, chronic back pain, diabetic neuropathy (nerve damage as a complication of diabetes), and arthritis. Supplements of tryptophan have also been reported to decrease a person's perception of pain. Conversely, drugs that interfere with serotonin production will increase one's sensitivity to pain.

People with chronic pain also tend to be depressed, understandably so, but the depression may not be simply a response to the disability and suffering. Since chronic pain and depression so often coincide, it is thought that lowered serotonin availability may be the common factor linking the two. Increasing serotonin availability will improve mood and pain tolerance; decreased serotonin availability will increase depression and increase pain sensitivity. Because decreased serotonin levels can also result in more impulsive and aggressive behavior, however, sometimes the reverse is seen. An aggressive, combative animal with low serotonin levels appears to be less sensitive to injury. For human beings troubled with depression, chronic pain, or both, increasing brain serotonin unquestionably has a positive impact.

Within the brain and spinal cord, serotonin acts to suppress pain signals. Endorphin release in the damaged or stressed tissue is thought to activate serotonin signals that diminish the pain message. In the rest of the nervous system, however, serotonin has actions that increase pain. As part of the inflammatory response, serotonin-rich platelets (the sticky blood cells that close a wound) pass out of the capillaries into the injured tissue. There the serotonin stimulates the release of bradykinin and substance P, two substances that irritate the nerves, increasing the local perception of pain. In one experiment involving some brave volunteers, serotonin applied directly to a blister increased the pain. This local effect of serotonin is less significant than its influence on pain awareness. Ultimately, it is the serotonin system in the brain that makes the command decision about how significant the pain is and how greatly it should occupy the brain's attention.

Chronic Pain: Is Serotonin the Body's Pain Thermostat?

Dr. William Willis at the University of Texas Medical Branch, Galveston, has studied the role of neurotransmitters in pain control, with a focus on serotonin. He investigated the theory that serotonin plays an important role in suppressing pain via signals sent from the brain's pain centers in the thalamus and brain stem to the spinal cord.

Dr. Willis confirmed that when the pain center of the thalamus is stimulated, increased amounts of serotonin are delivered into the pain pathways of the spinal cord. The amount of serotonin present in the spinal cord seemed to correspond to the degree of pain suppression. However, the amount never dropped to zero, leading him to theorize that serotonin could function as a pain thermostat. When levels in the spinal cord drop, he suggested, the pain system would be more responsive, and even slight injuries would be painful. When levels are increased, he proposed, you might get a general suppression of pain. Although this specific scenario is unproven, abundant evidence exists to support the view that serotonin in the brain's pain centers and in the spinal cord has an important role in moderating or suppressing pain awareness.

Serotonin and Headache

Migraine is often called vascular headache because the pain results in part from swelling of the blood vessels in the skull. Serotonin abnormalities are thought to influence these headaches in two different ways. Serotonin normally regulates blood vessel elasticity (expansion and contraction), acting mainly to constrict blood vessels. As blood vessels in the head expand in response to some irritant, they put pressure on surrounding tissues, causing pain. Also, they cause the release of serotonin into the tissues. As the next step, this serotonin causes the release of substance P from adjacent nerves, which increases the permeability of capillaries, so that substances leak into surrounding tissue as part of the inflammatory response to events that the body interprets as injury. This local fluid leakage (edema) includes an irritating and inflammatory chemical called bradykinin, which stimulates the pain-conducting nerves. To make matters worse, substance P is one of the most powerful facilitators of pain. It makes the pain-conducting nerve fibers more sensitive to the presence of bradykinin and to substance P itself. The vascular changes may be a source of pain, but sensitivity to pain has been greatly increased by the action of substance P and bradykinin.

Why does this happen? The release of these irritant chemicals from the nerve endings around blood vessels is normally controlled by a particular serotonin receptor. This specific serotonin receptor is defective in migraine sufferers, so that small, normally harmless triggers, such as certain foods, set off a series of changes in the blood vessels and nerves that result in pain.

Migraine, or "Sick Headache"

Migraines can be moderately to severely painful. A migraine attack usually lasts from four to twenty-four hours or longer. Most sufferers are not able to continue to function during an attack because movement, sound, and light can all intensify the pain. Withdrawing to a darkened bedroom to lie quietly or sleep is generally the sufferer's preferred strategy for dealing with the pain. In addition to throbbing one-sided head pain, the sufferer often has nausea and vomiting that can be as severe as the head pain—the reason for the name "sick headache." For some people the migraine attack will subside after vomiting.

About one in ten migraine sufferers will get strange symptoms called an aura in advance of a migraine. Most often these are disturbances in vision—twinkling lights, zigzag lines, or temporary loss of part of their field of vision. Tingling and numbness in part of the body can occur, and sometimes odd distortions in speech. With or without an aura, some migraine sufferers will have striking changes in mood—either depressed or elated—hours or a day or two before a migraine attack.

Migraine appears to be hereditary, and the evidence linking it to serotonin abnormalities is substantial. Measurements of serotonin levels in migraine sufferers suggest that the levels may go up and then dip suddenly before the migraine comes on, and mood often falls at the same time. Depression and migraine often coexist within the family, as well as within the same individual. In fact, a study by Michigan State researcher Naomi Breslau found that the risk of developing depression was more than three times higher for persons with migraine than persons with no history of migraine. Is this because suffering from migraine or any other chronic pain disorder causes someone to be depressed? Possibly, but the link between depression and migraine also works in reverse. In Dr. Breslau's study, persons with a history of major depression also had over three times the normal risk of developing migraine.

It does not seem that one condition causes the other; instead, both migraine and depression share the same underlying process, involving deficiencies in serotonin system functioning. Some studies suggest that the blood vessels of migraine sufferers may be much more sensitive to the effects of serotonin. Since serotonin is found in great abundance in the intestinal nervous system and it acts to cause the muscles of the gut to contract, it may also be involved in the nausea and vomiting many migraine sufferers experience during an attack.

The great majority of migraine sufferers, about 70 percent, are women. Although it can begin in childhood, the first migraine more commonly strikes during adolescence or early adulthood. In women, there is a clear relationship between migraine and hormones. Many women have their migraines triggered by falling estrogen levels in the days before menstruation. Birth control pills can make migraines worse; migraines often go away during pregnancy and after menopause.

A large range of dietary and environmental factors can trigger migraine, as well as fatigue or stress. Among the most common are foods containing high proportions of the amino acid tyramine (red wines, aged cheeses), foods containing nitrites (processed meats, such as hot dogs and cold cuts), and foods containing monosodium glutamate (MSG), which is included in a wide range of convenience or prepared foods, and is often listed on the ingredients simply as "natural flavors." Environmental factors include changes in weather, excessive heat or humidity, high altitudes, strong odors, and glaring or blinking lights. More information on identifying and avoiding migraine triggers is included in chapter 11.

Cluster Headache, the "Worst Pain in the World"

Unlike migraine and unlike many other serotonin-related problems, cluster headache largely afflicts men rather than women, in a ratio of about nine to one. Many people believe they have cluster headache because they experience migraine or tension headaches in a series or group. In fact, cluster headache is a uniquely severe type of headache in which the sufferer feels an extreme boring pain in and around one eye, like a red-hot poker being pressed into the socket. The eye—just that eye—will become very inflamed and may be teary or puffy. Often the nose will be congested in just the nostril on the same side as the affected eye. The headache will come on suddenly, often in the middle of a sound sleep, usually last a half hour or an hour, and then go away. There will be a series or cluster of attacks over the next few days or longer, then the headache will disappear for weeks or months before it strikes again. Cluster is also sometimes called "suicide headache" for its extreme pain, and "alarm clock headache" because it so often strikes during the middle of a sound sleep.

Although the patterns vary, cluster headache often strikes by the clock, at highly predictable times. During a cluster attack, the headaches may come at exactly the same time each day, or twice a day at twelve-hour intervals. In a ten-year study of four hundred patients, cluster headaches peaked in January and July, with the increase beginning seven to ten days after the winter and summer solstice. When the clocks were changed in the spring and fall between daylight savings and standard time, these patients had a decrease in attacks beginning seven to ten days after the "spring forward" or "fall back" time change. The punctuality and seasonal patterns suggest that cluster headache involves some abnormalities with the hypothalamus, the body's clock, which is responsible for regulating many basic functions, including sleep, appetite, body temperature, and other daily cycles. The hypothalamus is dense with serotonin receptors, as discussed in chapter 2, and serotonin takes a leading role in regulating these functions.

While migraine sufferers tend to crawl into bed and avoid moving, a person suffering a cluster headache will often become very agitated, pacing, running up and down, pounding on the walls in a fury that might be either a reaction to the horrible pain or a mood symptom that is part of the headache disorder. Unlike migraine, cluster headache has few clear triggers other than the seasonal changes described, but alcohol and altered sleeping patterns have been known to bring on cluster attacks. A substantial number of cluster headache sufferers are heavy drinkers and heavy smokers. Cutting back on both alcohol and nicotine is a good first step to managing the problem.

What About Everyday Tension Headache?

Tension or muscle-contraction headache most often feels like a vise or band pressing into the head. The pain may be in the front or back of the head, in the neck, or all three places at once. It is typically a steady, pressure-type pain, unlike the throbbing pain of migraine. It is generally less severe than migraine but can also come much more frequently. Some people have tension headache on a daily or near-daily basis.

Stress-related muscular tension in the neck and shoulders may contribute to bringing on these headaches or making them more severe. It may be that people prone to tension headache tend to express anger or worry physically by contracting the muscles of the neck or shoulder.

Even a few moments of muscle tension can be enough to trigger a pain response, which may not occur until hours later or even the next day. The muscle contraction temporarily reduces blood supply to the back of the head, and this reduced blood flow triggers a series of changes that will lead to pain. Despite the role of muscular tension or contraction as a headache trigger, these so-called tension headaches are now believed to result primarily from biochemical changes in the brain, possibly including the same serotonin system abnormalities found in migraine. Sufferers from chronic tension-type headaches also have been found to have abnormal serotonin system activity.

Some researchers doubt whether the distinction between headache types is actually meaningful, since many people have headaches that combine migraine and tension headache characteristics. This theory is partly supported by the fact that tension headaches are often relieved or prevented by the same serotonin-active medications that help with migraine.

Medication for Headache

People with occasional headache or infrequent migraines usually obtain good relief with over-the-counter pain remedies. Many chronic headache sufferers inadvertently make their problem much worse when they take these over-the-counter remedies on a daily or near-daily basis. A type of daily headache called analgesic rebound headache often results, in which the headache returns as the last dose of pain reliever wears off, creating a cycle of medication overuse and headache.

A variety of serotonin-active medications are successful in controlling chronic headache conditions. Ergot and ergotamine drugs act on the serotonin system. These include over-the-counter preparations such as Cafergot, Ercaf, and Migergot, as well as a very effective prescription medication, dihydroergotamine (available as Migranal intranasal spray or DHE-45 injection). Antidepressants can be quite helpful in reducing headache frequency and severity, regardless of whether the headache sufferer has any mood problems. The antidepressants apparently work by addressing the underlying serotonin abnormalities that trigger the headaches. By increasing serotonin availability, they may be also decreasing sensitivity to pain when a headache does occur.

Imitrex (sumatriptan) was developed to act directly on the serotonin receptor believed to be responsible for migraine. There are a lot of people out there with migraines, and Imitrex worked for them. This hugely successful drug was soon followed by an A-to-Z pharmacopoeia of me-too drugs, all new members of the triptan family: Axert (almotriptan), Relpax (eletriptan), Frova (frovatriptan), Amerge (naratriptan), Maxalt (rizatriptan), Zomig (zolmitriptan). There are some differences between these drugs in terms of the speed and duration of effects that may be meaningful for individual patients. However, there is no good evidence that any one drug is superior to another overall. Pharmaceutical companies often try to improve their market share by funding so-called phase IV postmarketing trials that compare their drug to the competition's. Often there are hidden biases in the design of the trial that favor the sponsor's drug. In any case, studies with disappointing outcomes may never get published—and certainly never get cited in the drug company's ad campaign! Don't let yourself be swayed by the ads into believing one drug is better than all the rest. Hopefully, your physician will know the pharmacology and will choose the drug most likely to work for you. (See the section on "Serotonin Syndrome" in chapter 2 for the potential risks of combining triptans with antidepressants.)

Pain on a Gut Level

Chronic indigestion, abdominal pain, irritable bowel syndrome, constipation, and diarrhea—these are hardly glamorous problems, no one likes to talk about them, but millions suffer from them. Serotonin abnormalities are now known to be underlying causes. Only 10 percent of serotonin is found in the brain; the remaining 90 percent is synthesized in the gut or intestines. Serotonin regulates the intestinal secretions and contractions (peristalsis) essential to digestion and excretion. As a result, abnormalities in gut serotonin functioning may lead to either constipation or diarrhea. Nausea and vomiting are regulated by serotonin centers in the brain stem that are in communication with the serotonin centers of the gut. Nausea and vomiting are essential safety mechanisms to deal with contaminated foods. (It's poison! Get rid of it! Fast!) But nausea (occasionally vomiting as well) can also be a very unpleasant feature of serotonin-related disorders such as PMS, migraine, and IBS—sometimes, even, the dominant and the most disabling symptom.

Serotonin, as we know, also modulates pain sensitivity both in the brain and body. Visceral hypersensitivity—an unpleasantly heightened awareness of intestinal sensations—is believed to underlie chronic abdominal pain complaints, making any cramping or bloating difficult or impossible to ignore. Often IBS first appears following a bout of stomach flu or food poisoning (gastroenteritis), and it may be that some combination of infection, genetic vulnerability, and life stress sets off a pattern of chronically disordered bowels and visceral hypersensitivity.

People with IBS in particular are at risk for other serotonin-related problems. A large population study published in *BMS Gastroenterology* in September of 2006 found that IBS sufferers have a 40 to 80 percent increase in the odds of also having migraine, depression, or fibromyalgia.

In fact, there is considerable symptom overlap among the pain conditions discussed in this chapter, inspiring spectrum disorder theories that these are not distinct conditions but differering manifestations of the same fundamental serotonin-related disorders. It has even been suggested that many cases of IBS might be alternatively diagnosed as fibromyalgia or migraine if the individual patient visited a rheumatologist or neurologist instead of a gastroenterologist.

Functional Dyspepsia: Medicalese for "We Don't Know What It Is"

Chronic or recurrent pain in the upper abdomen is often labeled "functional dyspepsia." In medical jargon, functional disorders are those for which no underlying structural or organic disease process can be identified. All the chronic pain conditions discussed in this chapter—migraine, cluster headache, irritable bowel syndrome, and fibromyalgia—are classified as functional disorders. It is an unfortunate term, since it often contains a hint, or an overt suggestion, that the condition is not quite real, that the patient is malingering or attention seeking or just whining. It is also a term that may say more about the limits of medical science than the nature of the illness. As imaging technologies have improved, there is increasingly firm evidence of real, if subtle, organic differences in the brains and biochemistry of the people with these disorders. It is not actually clear that functional dyspepsia is a distinct disorder from irritable bowel syndrome, since there is considerable symptom overlap, and the apparent difference in pain location may not be meaningful. Pain arising from disturbed functioning in the large intestine can be referred along the nerve pathways so that it is experienced in the upper abdomen instead. Many patients are somewhat arbitrarily diagnosed as having functional dyspepsia, IBS, or both. Treatment strategies are similar for both conditions.

Irritable Bowel Syndrome

IBS is characterized by recurrent or chronic abdominal discomfort (painful bloating or cramping) accompanied by diarrhea, constipation, or alternating episodes of both. Different serotonin system abnormalities are believed to account for the bowel symptoms and to direct the treatment options. The gut serotonin system is overactive for those who have diarrhea-predominant IBS—producing cramping and intestinal spasms, and frequent, watery stools. For constipation-predominant IBS, serotonin activity is reduced or deficient, resulting in intestinal bloating, stools that are difficult to pass, and sometimes severe constipation.

It is all too easy to imagine how the person with severe IBS might be doubted by family, friends, and doctors. Everyone gets an upset stomach now and then. Everyone has unpleasant visits to the bathroom—either undertaken at a quick run or as a prolonged stay. Implication: So what are you complaining about? What makes you different? Answer: The full spectrum of signs and symptoms associated with IBS is quite varied and complex. It can include insomnia, other sleep disturbances (longer REM sleep), changes in intestinal cell walls and secretions, abnormal urinary frequency and urgency, anxiety, depression, sexual problems (in women, painful intercourse), fibromyalgia, headaches, and chronic fatigue. Mild IBS may actually be quite common among men and women with other serotonin-related disorders. But IBS can be severe for a minority of patients. The diarrhea can be so sudden, extreme, and unpredictable that the sufferer is afraid to leave home.

People with IBS are finally getting a little respect for their embarrassing illness from researchers and physicians. Some of this attention stems from the pharmaceutical industry's keen interest in a potential market estimated (not quite credibly) at 60 million people in the United States alone! But family doctors as well as gastroenterologists are increasingly knowledgeable about IBS and sympathetic toward the patient complaining of chronic constipation or diarrhea and stomach pain. Unfortunately, there are limits, at this point, in what doctors have to offer as treatments.

A number of serotonin-active drugs have been tried for IBS. Serotonin receptor *agonists* (drugs that stimulate the serotonin system) have been used for constipation-predominant IBS, while serotonin receptor *antagonists* (drugs that block the receptor and so reduce serotonin activity) have been used for diarrhea-predominant IBS.

Thus far, the IBS-specific drugs that have reached the market have had limited efficacy and potentially severe side effects. With some of these drugs, the side effects may be difficult to recognize in a timely fashion, since they produce symptoms—such as intestinal pain and severe constipation—similar to those of the disorder itself. In particular, Lotronex (alosetron) was withdrawn after more than a hundred hospitalizations, fifty emergency surgeries, and at least seven deaths were linked to the drug. Following an FDA write-in campaign by patients, Lotronex was subsequently reintroduced with more restrictive labeling for IBS with severe diarrhea (women only). Old-fashioned tricyclic antidepressants, such as Anafranil or Norpramin, may be both safer and more effective for IBS. These drugs have general pain-relieving properties, and one of their more annoying side effects, constipation, can be a benefit for patients with diarrhea-predominant IBS.

Zelnorm (tegaserod) was developed to treat IBS with severe constipation (again women only—it is not effective for men). Although Zelnorm was statistically effective compared to a placebo in the studies that led to FDA approval, the success rate of this treatment is dismally low. At a 4 mg dose, it is effective in one in twenty patients and at a 12 mg dose in one in fourteen. There have also been worrying reports of side effects and complications with Zelnorm.

Surprisingly, one small but well-designed study (reported in the October 2005 issue of *Gut*) found that 3 mg of melatonin taken at bedtime provided pain relief for IBS sufferers with sleep disturbances. Oddly enough, the melatonin had no effect on sleep but did reduce abdominal pain and discomfort compared to placebo. It would be nice to have this study repeated and validated in a larger group of patients. In the meantime, given the few medical options available for people with bad IBS, a two-week trial of melatonin (3 mg at bedtime) is worth considering.

If you accept the pharmaceutical industry's estimate of the prevalence of IBS as 20 percent of the population, or 60 million people in the United States, then IBS obviously is not an illness for the vast majority of people with mild or occasional bowel symptoms. Rather, it is simply the way that their bodies deal with stress—in particular, perhaps, the stress of a lifestyle that is uncoupled from the traditional and natural rhythms of daytime (mostly outdoors) physical activity, followed by nighttime relaxation and sleep. Currently, lifestyle modification, including better diet, exercise, and relaxation and stress reduction techniques, are the safest and most effective long-term approaches to minimizing the pain and discomfort of IBS.

Pain Everywhere—Fibromyalgia

Fibromyalgia is characterized by widespread pain and by the presence of specific trigger points of muscle pain sensitivity located on the neck, shoulders, buttocks, knees, and elbows. As with so many other serotonin-related disorders, it is far more common in women than men, and it often overlaps with other conditions, including migraines or other chronic headaches, IBS, mood disorders (depression and anxiety), and insomnia. Because the diagnostic criteria are vague, many physicians have been skeptical that fibromyalgia is a genuine disorder, but evidence is now accumulating to demonstrate underlying biochemical differences in pain sensitivity and stress hormones in patients with fibromyalgia. The National Institute of Arthritis and Musculoskeletal and Skin Diseases (NIAMS), a division of the National Institutes of Health (NIH), has begun funding research in fibromyalgia to better understand its risk factors, causes, and treatment.

Studies have suggested that a number of nondrug or lifestyle approaches may ease pain and improve functioning, including aerobic exercise, relaxation therapy, biofeedback, and cognitive behavioral therapy. Because fibromyalgia often occurs in conjunction with serotonin-related conditions, a number of antidepressant therapies have been tried for fibromyalgia. The tricyclic antidepressants (Elavil, Anafranil, etc.), which have analgesic effects unrelated to their effects on mood, seem generally more effective for fibromyalgia than the SSRIs (Prozac, Zoloft, Paxil, etc.) Another option with some evidence of benefit is Flexeril (cyclobenzaprine), a muscle relaxant that is chemically similar to the tricyclic antidepressants.

Your Private Pain

You can say "look," "listen," or "feel this," and share a sight, sound, or texture with someone else. You cannot share the experience of pain because it is so private and so subjective. No one can ever know what someone else's pain is like. That is part of the mental distress for sufferers of chronic pain, who may feel doubted and misunderstood by both their family and their physicians, when something that is "just a headache" or "just an upset stomach" to others is overwhelmingly painful and incapacitating to them.

When the idea of low versus high pain thresholds first became popularized, many people immediately used it as a synonym for being weak versus being tough or brave. The idea really means that awareness of pain is under the control of a number of different neurotransmitters, including serotonin, endorphins, and substance P, among others. The threshold for pain depends on how the action of those various neurotransmitters is balanced, something that not only varies from individual to individual but from moment to moment.

An explanation for why pain awareness can vary so much has been offered by researchers Patrick Wall of University College, London, and Ronald Melzack of McGill University. Their "gate theory" of pain proposes that pain signals must pass through a number of gates as they move upward through the spinal cord into the brain. These gates are partially controlled by signals passing between the brain, spinal cord, and nerves in the areas experiencing the "hurt." For example, a slow-traveling pain sensation can be blocked at the gate by other sensations traveling on faster conducting nerves. When you instinctively rub a bruise or an aching forehead, you create a "distraction" that causes the nerves to report a second set of sensations that displace the pain signals, diminishing the sense of pain. The balance of serotonin, norepinephrine, endorphins, and other neurotransmitters is thought to have an important role in determining whether the pain signals get priority or are blocked by other messages saying, in effect, "It's no big deal—other stuff is more important."

Mood and activity can greatly affect the awareness of pain. A headache aches a great deal more when you are bored and frustrated than when you are distracted by conversation, chores, reading, or TV. An emergency or an urgent priority can suppress awareness of pain altogether. Athletes are often unaware of an injury or feel very little pain until after they leave the field. A phenomenon called "emergency analgesia" sometimes occurs on a battlefield or during a catastrophe as part of the body's adrenaline-fueled response to a crisis. People with terrible injuries are sometimes able to help comrades escape or are able to flee the scene themselves and collapse only after they have reached safety.

One of the most striking tales of emergency analgesia was told by David Livingstone, the nineteenth-century explorer of Africa. He was attacked by a lion, which sunk its teeth into his shoulder and brought him to the ground, shaking him as a house cat shakes a mouse. At that moment, he reports, he lost all sense of terror and pain, even though he remained conscious and perfectly aware of what was happening to him. He guessed that all animals might have a similar experience when attacked by a predator, "and if so, [it] is a merciful provision by our benevolent creator for lessening the pain of death."

Although the stress of an emergency can activate the body's pain control system, stress more generally acts to increase or even to cause pain. We often think of stress simply in terms hectic schedules and multiple demands on our time. In fact, stress can be anything that disrupts the body's normal functions and cycles, including drugs, alcohol, chemicals, sleep deprivation, noise, and infections. And pain itself, of course, is perhaps the greatest stress of all.

The placebo effect, discussed in chapter 4, is often taken as evidence that the pain is not genuine. In fact, very real and debilitating pain can be relieved by a placebo treatment when the sufferer is determined to get or hopeful of getting relief. During the Korean conflict, an army surgeon suddenly experienced severe pain from appendicitis just as a large number of wounded were brought into the hospital base. He knew he could safely postpone his own surgery for a few hours while he tended to the wounded, so long as he had some relief from the pain. He ordered a nurse to give him an injection of morphine, and he felt pain-free moments later, which allowed him to continue to work. A week or so later, after his appendix had been removed and he had recovered, he happened to check the nurse's log. It read: "Doctor _____ was very agitated, so I judged best to give him saline rather than morphine." A placebo had completely relieved the agonizing pain of an infected appendix!

The dramatic success that placebo treatments can sometimes have points to the power of the sufferer's mind and mood to make the pain worse or to make the pain better. What we know about serotonin's roles in improving mood and reducing pain strongly suggests that we are not merely the helpless victims of our physical and emotional pain. Serotonin-enhancing exercise and positive coping techniques to improve mood will also improve a person's pain threshold by drawing on the combined effects of serotonin and endorphins.

It is worth pointing out here that the opposite is also true. The *nocebo effect* is a tendency to become ill in response to negative expectations or fears. (For people interested in words, *nocebo* is Latin for "I will cause pain," while *placebo* means "I will please.") For example, medical students are notorious for developing symptoms of a disease they are studying. Anxious fears about one's health can bring on symptoms of heart attack or other disease, as discussed in chapter 6. Feelings of fear and helplessness during an attack of chronic pain, such as headache or arthritis, can create stress and tension that will make the pain worse. As another form of the nocebo effect, some people will develop very unusual or severe side effects to drugs they are uncomfortable about taking.

Chronic Pain and Relationships

For people with chronic pain conditions, managing relationships can be as great a problem as managing the pain itself. Family outings and social engagements must be canceled when a sudden pain flare-up strikes, so many sufferers must limit how much they try to do socially. Friends and acquaintances are likely not to understand why a headache or stomachache gets in the way of a dinner engagement, and repeated cancellations may cancel the friendship.

Closer to home, sufferers may find that their family's understanding, sympathy, and patience diminish over time when they don't "get better." This is all the more the case if the doctors consulted focus on finding a physical or organic cause of pain, then withdraw their interest and concern after they determine that the pain is "benign." If an injury brought on the first bout of pain—such as a concussion that results in headaches or back pain—both the family and the family doctor may have an unstated timetable for recovery. If the pain continues undiminished, they will suspect that the sufferer is malingering, just to enjoy the attention and the sympathy, even though the attention and sympathy may have largely disappeared!

Of course, just the opposite may happen, and often does. The crisis created by the injury and the pain brings the family closer together. They rally to take care of the sufferer, and a child or spouse who may have been taken a bit for granted is suddenly the focus of the family's life together. Perhaps the intimacy had drained out of a basically stable marriage: A too-busy, work-obsessed husband may have rarely touched his wife or expressed affection. He becomes much more supportive and involved in response to her pain and disability, which elicit a tenderness he hasn't shown in years. Or if there were problems in the marriage, the mother and father may be brought together by their anxiety and concern for a daughter who begins having excruciating migraines. Even a small child can perceive that not only is she getting much more love and attention, but her parents aren't fighting anymore because of her illness. She then has powerful unconscious motivation to continue to suffer. The same can be true with other relationships. Perhaps you only called your father once a week or so before he injured his back. Now you feel worried and guilty, so you come by or at least call every day because his recovery has been painful and slow.

Could you and your family be unconsciously perpetuating the pain by showing more love and attention during sickness than during health? Ask yourself the following questions:

- Are we closer now than we were before the pain?
- Have our lives become focused on preventing the pain and taking care of the family member with the pain?
- Are intimacy, affection, and "quality time" offered more often when the sufferer is in pain than when he or she is pain free?

If you answer yes to any two or to all three questions, you should consider whether these family behaviors might be perpetuating the pain by rewarding it. This does not mean that the pain is any less real or horrible or that the sufferer is seeking attention—just that everyone in the relationship has become invested in the pain's continuing rather than in its getting better. In psychological terms, being in pain is "reinforced," rewarded, or supported—in effect, encouraged—while being pain free is not! This situation is unfair and detrimental to the well-being of the sufferer as well as to everyone else in the family. If someone in your family suffers from chronic pain, try examining your own behavior to be sure you are being truly helpful. The following strategies can guide you:

- When the pain strikes, express sympathy, provide any *necessary* assistance, then give the sufferer some privacy. You really cannot help.
- When the pain is absent or is down to tolerable levels, reward the sufferer with your appreciation and attention. Make these pain-free intervals your quality time together.

These ways of interacting with the sufferer will not, of course, cure chronic pain. But they will help to ensure that the pain isn't being perpetuated by both the sufferer's and the family's *need* for the pain as a vehicle for intimacy.

Often family and friends try to respond to the problem with a variety of ideas and advice meant to be helpful such as, "Get some exercise—you'll feel better," "Try getting some sleep," "You're not eating right," or "Take some vitamin C." Although all these statements may be true, repeating them constantly does not help the sufferer. The hidden message dismisses the significance of the pain and criticizes the sufferer for what he or she has or hasn't done. The urge to give advice should be resisted.

At the same time, the sufferer should not expect to be continually listened to when the message, even to those closest and most sympathetic, seems like a broken record. No one truly can understand or feel someone else's pain. The best listeners and realistic advice givers are fellow sufferers.

There are organized support groups for many chronic pain disorders. Support groups are not helpful if they become dominated by negativity and venting. A skilled group leader works to focus the group on sharing positive coping strategies and experiences.

Pain Free and Drug Free

Pain-relieving medications (either analgesics or narcotics for severe pain) are generally safe and effective for short-term treatment of acute pain resulting from an injury, surgery, or a disease that runs its course then goes away. For chronic pain—either pain that is continually present or recurs on a regular basis—long-term dependence on medication may be necessary as a last resort. It is not the preferred choice of most sufferers and their physicians. There are a variety of excellent nondrug treatments for pain. Even if you require medication to control the pain of headache, IBS, fibromyalgia, or arthritis, you may be able to reduce both the pain and the need for medication by following the nutritional guidelines and practicing special exercise and relaxation techniques covered in this book.

Biofeedback is a pain reduction technique that has been shown to be effective in study after study. Basically, biofeedback teaches you how to become aware of changes in your body that generally are automatic and involuntary—such as blood flow and muscle tension. With biofeedback, you learn to detect and reverse your body's stress responses, which can bring on or aggravate pain. Biofeedback requires a trained practitioner and special equipment that detects your body's changes and uses them as feedback to focus and direct your efforts to relax. Tension headache sufferers are often trained to relax using biofeedback equipment that measures the electrical activity in head and neck muscles, which is a measure of how contracted or relaxed the muscles are. Another common system uses a monitor to detect the temperature of the finger—a shortcut way to measure the level of stress or tension in your body. By learning how to raise the temperature of your finger at will, you are able to relax muscles and indirectly control or block stress-related biochemical changes in your nervous system. Biofeedback can also be used to reach a state called deep relaxation, in which blood flow is stabilized throughout the body and the electrical activity of the muscles and of the brain is at its minimum—an "alpha wave" state corresponding to that achieved by advanced meditation techniques. Biofeedback is an excellent choice for someone who is uncomfortable with relying on medication but is not able to obtain adequate pain control from self-training in relaxation exercises.

6

Worry and Nitpicking: Anxiety, Obsessive-Compulsive Behavior

Anxiety, like depression, can be a natural response to a hostile environment. Without anxiety, and the hyperalert state that usually accompanies it, we would be much less successful at driving on icy roads, avoiding injuries, or protecting the safety of our children and our home. A mild anxiety-like state—such as a nagging sense of discontent or discomfort with the way things are—can be a great spur to moving forward with our lives and accomplishing new things. Anxiety is always unpleasant, yet as a response to real threats and obstacles, it helps us to survive and thrive.

Often, though, anxiety is out of proportion to the threat. One person might worry obsessively over a rumor that the company is being bought, even though there is minimal chance her job would be affected. Another might be overwhelmed with fear and anxiety if his daughter doesn't come home on time, or doesn't call when she said she would. This kind of anxiety robs us of our sleep, our enjoyment of life, and sometimes our health.

Can't Stop Worrying

Do you worry, not just sometimes, but on an ongoing basis, for weeks at a time? Are you always fearful that something will happen to your family, your job, your home, or your health? Does any little event—your kid's bad report card; an odd, fleeting pain in your chest; or a negative response from your boss—send you into a tailspin? When some little thing happens that seems to confirm your worst fears, do you lose sleep and have physical symptoms, such as stomach upset, muscular tension, or a pounding heart? Do other people say, "You worry too much; relax, take it easy"?

If yes, you may well have a significant problem with anxiety, but the advice to relax is unlikely to help you. Chronic anxiety is now believed to result from biochemical changes that include abnormalities in the neurotransmitters norepinephrine and serotonin. You have constant anxiety because of these abnormalities, not because there is something fundamentally wrong with either your character or your life. If you won the lottery tomorrow, six months later you would probably start worrying about finances again, and if you took a job as a mattress tester you might still feel anxious about doing well enough at your work.

Norepinephrine, mentioned already in chapter 2, is part of the body's stress response. It serves to give you the energy and alertness to deal with a crisis. Serotonin has an important role in moderating or dampening that "Danger! Danger!" red alert that goes off in our heads when we are startled, intimidated, confused, or just plain anxious. As we deal with stressful events and with the sheer complexity of everything happening around us, norepinephrine and serotonin are important to how our brain sorts through events and sensations, dismissing some as trivial, paying attention to others as important for our welfare. If the norepinephrine system is overactive or overresponsive, while the serotonin system is underactive or imbalanced, we are at risk for suffering from unnecessary worrying and from full-blown anxiety disorders.

Stress, Anxiety, and the Body

You may remember hearing about the medical theory that the anxious, controlling, obsessive type A personality is more prone to high blood pressure and heart disease. First proposed decades ago, this theory is not considered proven beyond doubt, but many studies since that time have supported it. A Harvard Medical School study that monitored the health of over two thousand men for thirty-two years found that middle-aged men who gave yes answers to two or more of the following questions were at increased risk of sudden, fatal heart attacks:

1. Do strange people or places make you afraid?
2. Are you considered a nervous person?
3. Are you constantly keyed up and jittery?
4. Do you often become suddenly scared for no good reason?
5. Do you often break out in a cold sweat?

For the men answering yes to two or more of these questions, the risk of dying from heart disease was more than three times higher, while the risk of sudden death was increased almost sixfold, compared to men who answered no to all five questions.

For anyone who has ever had an anxiety attack, the relationship of anxiety to high blood pressure and heart attack is not hard to understand. Acute anxiety or fear will cause the heart to pound and the pulse to race. Blood pressure does go up. Someone who is already at risk might well reach dangerously high blood pressure during moments of added stress or tension.

Quiet, chronic worrywarts know that they worry. People with anxiety sometimes aren't aware that what they are feeling is anxiety because the physical symptoms may be much more obvious than the worrying. For some, anxiety is too wimpy to acknowledge. Instead, they focus on the physical symptoms, which can be very alarming:

- Shortness of breath, asthma, hyperventilating (overbreathing)
- Rapid heartbeat, heart palpitations, chest pain
- Sweating
- Lightheadedness, dizziness, faintness
- Tingling, weakness, or numbness in arms and legs; headache
- Stomach pain, nausea, vomiting, diarrhea, cramps, frequent urination

They may be quite aware of feeling anxious, but assume it is the result rather than the cause of the frightening physical symptoms.

As a serotonin-related problem, anxiety has a variety of mood, food, motivation, and sleep symptoms, in addition to the physical ones already listed:

- Keyed-up feeling, tense inside
- Sense of impending doom
- Worrying about trifles
- Difficulty falling asleep or early A.M. awakening
- Difficulty concentrating
- Changed appetite
- Sexual problems

Biology, Not Character

The painful and frightening symptoms of an acute anxiety attack have a significant function in the body. They are part of what is called the fight-or-flight response, which is the way people and animals marshal their energies to respond to danger. If you are running from a lion or meeting an enemy in battle this hyperalert "all systems go" response helps you meet the challenge to your physical survival. Of course, when you are lying awake in bed at 3 A.M., wondering how you will make your mortgage payments if you are laid off, it is not at all helpful. A racing heart, darting eyes, and twitching muscles do not help us cope with a much more abstract sense of danger and alarm.

The folk wisdom that chronic worry and jumpiness are all "nerves" is surprisingly close to the target. People subject to anxiety attacks of one type or another are thought to have a hypersensitive nervous system that responds too readily to perceived threats or emergencies. During this fight-or-flight response, the body and brain release a flood of energizing and activating hormones, including adrenaline and cortisone, and the neurotransmitter norepinephrine. Your heart and pulse rates quicken; your breathing becomes shallow and rapid; muscles tense for action; and the liver releases a surge of stored sugar to give you the energy to meet your challenge.

An anxious human, like an anxious animal, will experience nervous and muscular tension, accompanied by a jumpy, excessive sensitivity to sights and sounds that is noticeable to others. People prone to anxiety tend to scan a room with their eyes, unconsciously on the lookout for danger. They may also startle much more readily than others, flinching at an unexpected noise or encounter. These are excellent instincts to have in a jungle or savannah that is heavily populated with predators, but not when walking down a safe city street or stepping into a supervisor's office.

Often the person who develops disabling physical symptoms of anxiety is one who has rigorously and almost heroically avoided feeling anxious in response to some major stress or life transition. When anxious thoughts and feelings intruded, the response might have been to throw oneself into work or other activities—perhaps out of a sense that anxiety was weak or perhaps from a fear that there would be no escaping or controlling the anxiety once it was let out into the open. People who are less "in control" often handle anxiety more easily.

Sad and Worried

Chronic anxiety not only gets you sick, it gets you down. Depression very commonly accompanies anxiety. The relationship between the two moods is complex. Feeling one may put you at increased risk of the other. Prolonged anxiety may lead to depression by producing a type of emotional and physical exhaustion. Depression and anxiety can be difficult to tell apart, even for experts. Guilty and pessimistic feelings characterize depression, while the anxious person fears disaster without necessarily feeling bad about himself or herself or life in general. Anxiety is usually a state of painful agitation, while depression can involve either agitation or a slowing down of responsiveness and energy. Both mood problems bring sleep and appetite changes with them. Specific antidepressants are often effective in relieving anxiety, while others are not. As covered in chapter 11, exercise can have major benefits in relieving both the physical tension and the mental preoccupation of chronic anxiety.

Doctor, I Have These Awful Symptoms...

It has been estimated that as many as one-quarter of all visits to the family physician are because of pain for which no organic or physical cause can be found. Pain can be a symptom of anxiety or depression, perhaps due to defects in the serotonin pain regulation system, or it can be an indirect by-product of mood and stress. The stress response of acute anxiety or chronic worrying can produce gastrointestinal symptoms such as diarrhea and cramps; the muscle tension can bring on back and neck pain and tension headache.

Because so many of the signs of anxiety are physical, many sufferers spend much time and money seeing specialists and getting tested, with no results. They may be unaware of their feelings of stress, anxiety, and doom, or think that the emotional distress results from the physical symptoms, rather than the other way around. Sometimes physicians also focus on physical signs, and when they are unable to detect an underlying disease, dismiss the patient with "It's nothing but your nerves; don't worry so much" or "I can't find anything wrong with you; maybe you need a vacation—or a therapist." This feedback is far from helpful or reassuring, since the sufferer feels belittled or doubted, and the underlying biochemical causes have not been addressed or treated.

Performance Anxiety and Other Trials of the Nerves

Almost everyone has at least minor problems with stage fright or performance anxiety. In one survey that asked American adults about their greatest fears, public speaking came in number one—ahead of cancer! Fear of taking tests, examination nerves, is another common form of performance anxiety. It can persist all through adult life in the form of recurring school anxiety dreams, such as the one about that course you signed up for and never attended, forgetting all about it until right now, the day of the final exam.

A moderate degree of performance anxiety is quite helpful in focusing your concentration and motivation. Without a little bit of anxiety, you would not prepare quite so hard for that important meeting or sales call, and you would not be so attentive to the details. Too much anxiety, of course, has just the opposite effect. Flooded by our fear, we cannot think, cannot speak. People who suffer from performance anxiety often assume it is easier for others. In fact, many veteran performers, such as college lecturers, actors, and musicians, approach each public appearance with some degree of shakiness, sweating, nausea, and butterflies. Many musicians rely, more or less secretly, on beta blockers such as Inderal (propranolol) to relieve the pounding heart, shakiness, and nausea that might otherwise interfere with their performance. Of course, if the performance anxiety stems from having a highly self-critical and perfectionistic personality, a blood pressure medication can do nothing to relieve the misery that results from obsessing over a single wrong note or mistimed phrasing.

Social Jitters

～

You get an invitation to a party or a wedding. You're pleased and flattered—of course you'll come. As the day rolls round, however, you begin to dread the occasion. Will other people you know be there? Suppose no one wants to talk to you, and you're left sitting in a corner alone? What if you wear the wrong clothes? Everyone will look at you and wonder what's the matter with you! You go, feeling butterflies in your stomach, as nervous as before a final exam in college. Or maybe you actually do feel so sick you decide to stay home.

Social phobia or social anxiety is very common. Vast numbers of attractive and intelligent people face social occasions with a hidden dread of making a fool of themselves. For some this fear is so disabling that they reject invitations and are unable to date, even though they hate to be alone. People who can deal comfortably with everyone in a business setting may become totally tongue-tied and humiliated when they try to hold a conversation with someone they find sexually attractive. If they force themselves to try, they may feel so self-conscious that they come off as cold, aloof, unreachable. Puzzled friends say, "What got into you? You're usually so much fun!" Many people are able to control their nervousness well enough so that they can go out socially, but they must cover their anxiety and discomfort by frequent trips to the bar. Social anxiety is a major motive for drinking too heavily at parties and clubs.

Social phobias can take a number of other forms. Some people have great difficulty eating in public or using a public restroom. A dread of looking foolish or being put down may keep them from asking directions when they are lost or returning defective merchandise to a store. Anxiety about writing while someone is watching—for fear your hand will tremble and it will be noticed—can make it hard for people to handle everyday transactions like writing checks or signing credit card bills.

Often the person with social phobia was shy as a small child but then socialized with no real problems until adolescence, when social anxiety usually begins. As with other forms of anxiety, physical symptoms— blushing, sweating, throat constriction and choking sensation, and mental confusion—make the problem worse, since the sufferer dreads other people noticing his or her discomfort and nervousness. In surveys, nearly half of all Americans describe themselves as shy, yet every sufferer from stage fright, dating anxiety, examination nerves, or job interview jitters feels that he or she is all alone in a world of cool, poised, never-at-a-loss sophisticates.

Just One Thing in the World

Phobias can be highly specific. You can handle just about anything with aplomb that gives other people jitters—public speaking, rush-hour traffic, rough neighborhoods—but an insect buzzing around your head or crawling up the wall fills you with terror. You can hardly leave the city in the summer, and you feel almost sick when someone comes back from Florida and describes the size of the cockroach they saw in their hotel.

Someone else might have a phobic fear of cats or dogs . . . or swallowing pills . . . the sight of blood . . . knives . . . bridges . . . being in tall buildings. Virtually anything can be the object of a phobia, even water or light.

Friends and family often try to help the phobic sufferer get past the fear by, for example, bringing a cat into the room and trying to get the sufferer to pet it—"It won't hurt you. Look, it just wants to be friends." Usually the phobic individual makes a brave but unsuccessful effort to be convinced, and may almost pass out from relief when the cat is finally taken out of the room. This "face-your-fear" approach is in fact the technique that experts use with good success to cure phobia, only they proceed much more slowly. The sufferer is first asked to visualize a cat. If symptoms of anxiety arise, reassurance is given that the symptoms are harmless and won't bring on a heart attack or seizure. The next step might be to write the word "cat" over and over again, then to look at a picture of a cat while practicing deep breathing and other calming exercises. Bringing a cat into the same room is the final stage of the gradated exposure, or desensitization, approach. It might well take hours or repeated sessions before the phobic sufferer is finally able to touch the cat without fear.

There are well-structured programs (often sponsored by airlines) to help people deal with one of the most common of all phobias, fear of flying. Somewhere between 10 and 40 percent of the general population are either white-knuckle fliers or never fliers. Hospitals sometimes have programs to help people deal with phobias about blood and needles that may prevent them from donating blood or getting needed medical care.

Phobias may begin in childhood, after a frightening encounter with, for example, a dog, spider, or snake. Well-intentioned parental teaching that guns, germs, fire, and knives are dangerous can also stir phobic fears in children who are biologically at risk. Phobias may fade away in adolescence and then resurface in adulthood during a period of stress or major life change.

Panic Attacks

Most people have felt some form of stage fright—the sweaty palms, pounding heart, tension, dry mouth, and tightness in the throat that you experience before public speaking, an important meeting, or a confrontation of some sort. Sufferers from panic attacks have these symptoms come over them from out of the blue. Acute panic feels awful. There is physical tension, heart palpitations, nausea, sweating, choking sensation, struggling for breath, along with a sense of overwhelming dread. There can be strange feelings of alienation from your body, or that your body is coming apart. The person suffering a sudden panic attack often fears passing out, going crazy, or having a heart attack. Those fears can then magnify the symptoms even more.

Panic attacks are usually associated with some crisis, stress, or life change. You've just moved to a strange city to begin a new job. You're happy about the change and feel no more than the nervousness anyone would feel in a strange place. As you are getting settled into your new life, you start to have symptoms of some terrible disease. In the supermarket or on the way to work, you start to choke, your heart pounds, your vision swims. You are barely able to get out of the store or pull over to the curb. The strange attack passes but it comes again, first in the same situations and then unpredictably. You don't know what to do. You see a doctor, but all the tests are negative. Hopefully, the doctor will diagnose the problem as a panic attack and provide reassurance or referral to take care of the problem. Panic attacks respond very well to behavioral approaches to helping the victim understand that the symptoms are benign and controllable.

Sometimes panic attacks do not have such an obvious trigger as a new job or other big change. Sometimes a single bad day or bad week of slightly greater than average pressure and strain will bring on the initial attack. The unexplained terror of that first attack can then bring on repeated attacks.

Fear of Fear Itself

Moderate anxiety helps spur us to find a solution to the problem confronting us. Severe anxiety can have just the opposite effect. The feeling is so terrible that we do anything to avoid the person, place, or thing that provokes anxiety. Rather than master our fear of making presentations or socializing with new people, we limit our work and recreation to escape those situations, missing out on opportunities to enrich our lives. This avoidance then makes the problem seem all the more terrible and insurmountable. The avoidance escalates the fear, along with producing a powerful conviction of failure and helplessness.

For example, after repeated panic attacks, the sufferer usually tries to avoid doing anything that might trigger another. If the attacks came while driving on a busy expressway, he or she might start taking back roads to and from work. Or if the panic hit while stuck in a crowd in a busy department store, the person might avoid crowds or avoid shopping except during off-hours. If the attacks continue, the sufferer will make further restrictions—not driving more than a few miles from home, for example, or even not driving at all. The need to avoid another attack, and the fear of losing control completely or having a heart attack, can lead to a generalized fear of public places, called agoraphobia.

People suffering from agoraphobia may be unable to leave home because of their anxiety. More commonly, they can carry out a mostly normal life so long as they avoid any situation in which they feel trapped. Elevators, airplanes, and crowded rooms can bring on a terrible fear of having a panic attack in public, and that fear can be all it takes to precipitate the attack. People with agoraphobia will scan a room or building as they enter, noting the available exits. At a party, restaurant, meeting, or lecture, they will stay as close to the door as they can manage.

The "Anxious" Circle

Chronic or low-level worrying is likely to produce back pain, neck pain, tension headache, or gastrointestinal symptoms such as diarrhea. Unpleasant as these may be, acute anxiety produces much more terrifying physical sensations—a racing pulse, swimming vision, gasping for breath, pounding heart, even chest pain that radiates into the arm like a real heart attack. If some momentary terror inspired this fight-or-flight response— say, the sudden appearance of a stranger behind you on a dark street—the sufferer can usually calm down, recognizing the physical response everyone has to a sudden shock or fear. But when a panic attack comes out of the blue, the victim has no way of understanding the symptoms except as a heart attack or some other catastrophic illness. This fear, of course, makes the symptoms intensify. If your heart just skipped a beat at your first moment of alarm, now it's pounding as though it's going to jump out of your chest!

On a milder scale, the same vicious circle occurs with performance anxiety and social phobia. You are particularly afraid of stammering or of blushing, thereby drawing people's attention and letting everyone know about your self-consciousness. Then this fear itself causes your throat to constrict so that you have trouble speaking, and your blood rushes to your skin, exposing your embarrassment. Your fears come true, confirming themselves, in a self-fulfilling cycle.

Anxiety, Serotonin, and Drugs

As you might expect, serotonin-active drugs, such as Prozac, Paxil, Zoloft, and BuSpar (buspirone), are a mainstay of medical treatment for severe anxiety. BuSpar is an antianxiety medication that acts on a particular serotonin receptor, and it can also relieve any accompanying symptoms of depression.

The specific serotonin defects involved in anxiety are still not yet well understood, in part because what we call anxiety may actually take different forms. A generalized chronic anxiety is quite different from panic attacks, and drugs effective for one are often much less successful in treating the other. Some of the uncertainty stems from the fact that we don't yet know how antianxiety drugs work. The serotonin-enhancing SSRI drugs (Zoloft, Prozac, etc.) often worsen anxiety during the initial treatment phase. BuSpar's short-term effect is to reduce serotonin activity involving a specific receptor, yet with extended treatment it seems to increase serotonin activity. It does not begin to relieve anxiety symptoms until around the third week of treatment. Since SSRI drugs like Prozac that increase serotonin availability throughout the brain are often effective in relieving anxiety with prolonged treatment, it does seem that the overall effect of serotonin is to reduce anxious feelings. These antianxiety effects are believed to be related to serotonin's ability to decrease norepinephrine system activity, quelling the high-adrenaline fight-or-flight response. It may be the case that a combination of low serotonin activity and high norepinephrine activity is needed to produce acute anxiety or panic.

There are many types of anxious moods and feelings, and serotonin activity in some parts of the brain may actually contribute to them. For example, serotonin activity is important for inhibiting impulsive or inappropriate behavior—making individuals more wary and cautious in the presence of a real threat or risk. Whether that serotonin-based cautiousness is experienced as self-control or as fearfulness is something we don't yet know. One view holds that people who are excessively cautious, inhibited, and perfectionistic have an overactive serotonin system, resulting in *too much* impulse control. Yet these same people often have signs of depression and will loosen up in response to a medication like Zoloft or Prozac that increases serotonin availability throughout the brain. It may be that serotonin's overall function is to control inappropriate or excessive responses in general, including excessive fearfulness.

Recent evidence from animal studies indicates that different types of serotonin receptors in different parts of the brain have distinct roles in modulating anxiety and the fight-or-flight response to stressful or frightening situations. For example, the amygdala is a region of the brain crucial for learning from painful or stressful experiences of the "once burned, twice shy" variety. Increasing serotonin levels in the amygdala produces anxious responses in animals. In contrast, increasing serotonin levels in another portion of the brain known as the PAG (short for periaqueductal gray matter, a region that modulates response to pain and danger) decreases fearful responses in animals. Some researchers theorize that serotonin release in the PAG restrains a panicky response, whereas in the amygdala serotonin release may act to increase the "what-if-ing" or anticipatory worrying of generalized anxiety. The complex dual role of serotonin in modulating the anxious response—increasing or decreasing it—likely explains why serotonin-active drugs are a less effective treatment overall than cognitive behavioral therapy.

Early in the last century, drug treatment for anxiety relied on barbiturates, which are addictive sedatives. They did not actually treat anxiety; they only drugged the person so he or she was unable to concentrate on anxiety-producing preoccupations until the sedating effects wore off. The first tranquilizer, Miltown (meprobamate), was introduced in the 1950s. It proved to be a spectacularly popular drug, since it appeared to relax and calm people without putting them to sleep. Further study showed that it was just as sedative and addicting as the barbiturates—but people liked what it did!

The next drugs to be introduced as antianxiety treatments were the benzodiazepines, such as Valium (diazepam) and Xanax (alprazolam), which are still in use today. They successfully relieve feelings of anxiety, and the mild mental impairment they cause usually does not interfere with everyday activities. Since anxious people are often insomniacs, the mild sedating effects are generally a benefit. These new drugs were very well received by a nation of anxious people, and their apparent safety led doctors to prescribe them freely to anyone complaining of mild anxiety or insomnia or just vague problems with coping. In 1975, U.S. pharmacists filled one hundred million prescriptions for Valium! Valium was the "cures what ails you" all-purpose panacea.

However, the benzodiazepines are addicting, though not as severely as barbiturates, and they can cause death or coma when combined with alcohol abuse. Concerns with public safety and with widespread drug dependency led to more conservative prescribing practices, and these drugs are now recommended only for short-term relief of acute anxiety, followed by a trial of one of the antidepressants (e.g., Effexor, Paxil, Zoloft, or Prozac) approved for the specific anxiety disorder.

When first introduced, there was not much understanding of how Valium and other benzodiazepines acted on the brain and nervous system to reduce anxiety. It has since been discovered that these drugs interact with specific receptors on nerve cells that have been named "benzodiazepine receptors" in their honor. Apparently, the brain has its own Valium-like chemicals that may act to calm or control anxious feelings, but the normal, drug-free role of these receptors is not yet well understood. These benzodiazepine receptors are present in the nervous system of the gut in great abundance, and it is thought that they may play a role in mood responses to eating. Some evidence suggests that these "benzodiazepine receptors" and a specific subtype of serotonin receptor (5-HT_{1A}) are malfunctioning in persons with anxiety disorders.

Because anxiety has such powerful self-reinforcing or self-perpetuating physical symptoms, some drugs can cause or relieve anxiety by acting on the body rather than the brain. As mentioned earlier, a quick-fix approach to the treatment of performance anxiety is to provide the sufferer with a supply of beta blockers, a medication that lowers blood pressure. Taken in advance of an anxiety-producing situation, the beta blocker will prevent the physical symptoms of anxiety, potentially giving the individual the confidence to carry him or her through the occasion. Similarly, drugs that cause physical symptoms resembling those of panic will bring on all the emotions of anxiety in a person who is prone to anxiety attacks. Someone not troubled with anxiety is more likely to separate the physical manifestations of fear from fear itself. Even as familiar a drug as caffeine can cause "coffee nerves" that sometimes include dramatic physical symptoms such as racing pulse, sweating, shaking, and faintness. Common over-the-counter drugs containing caffeine and other stimulants, such as cold remedies and diet pills, can also produce anxiety symptoms or even an actual panic attack. The same is true for abused stimulants such as amphetamines and cocaine. One of the simplest and best of the good-sense approaches to controlling anxiety is to cut down on caffeine and any other stimulants in your diet.

Of course, the oldest and most popular antianxiety drug of all is alcohol. Virtually everyone who touches the stuff has experienced its soothing effects on jangled nerves and tension. People with serious problems with anxiety are prone to have serious problems with alcohol, and vice versa. Although alcoholics almost always prove to have some underlying anxiety disorder, alcohol dependency also involves problems of impulse control. Alcohol abuse is covered in chapter 7.

Obsessions, Compulsions

The word "obsession" has romantic and poetic associations, enough to qualify it as the name of a perfume. For someone who suffers from an obsessive fear or compulsion, there is not much glamour involved. As a medical condition, obsessive-compulsive disorder, or OCD, is considered to be a form of anxiety. People who have some severe compulsive ritual, such as washing their hands a hundred times a day, are usually quite rational. They know the ritual is excessive and unreasonable. It's just that they feel terrible anxiety whenever they attempt to stop. The ritual itself eases their anxiety. We can easily recognize the feeling. Of course we know there's almost zero chance that we actually left a stovetop burner turned on. But if we check it once more before leaving the house, we know we won't worry about it while we're out.

Some obsessive-compulsive behavior is minor and quite common— double-checking that the doors and windows are locked, that the oven is off, or that you turned off the headlights after parking your car. How many people check to see if their letter dropped down the slot into the mailbox? Do you have a nervous habit when you're stressed, such as biting your nails? Let's have a show of hands!

Obsessive, detail-oriented people are essential to many professions. You wouldn't like to think that the engineer running the nuclear power plant twenty miles from your home, the accountant preparing your tax returns, or the surgeon taking out your gall bladder were happy-go-lucky types who shrugged off problems and fudged when they didn't know the correct procedures. Obsessions become troubling to others and to the sufferer when they seriously intrude on daily life. For example, worrying so much about your home, despite all your double-checking, that you cannot enjoy a weekend away; or, being so concerned about germs that you cannot bring yourself to use a public restroom, or can do so only if you wash your hands over and over again. Some people appear carefree and fearless, yet carry an invisible burden of obsession, ruminating on problems and what-if fears that they know aren't realistic yet they can't turn off.

An obsession is generally a recurring thought or theme, such as a fear or a suspicion that you are contaminated, or that you have inadvertently harmed someone, say by running them over with your car. Obsessions can be exhausting and debilitating all by themselves, since the thoughts are persistent, uncontrollable, and intrusive. An obsession can motivate a compulsion, such as washing your hands or stopping the car and repeatedly checking to make sure the bump in the road was a pothole, not a baby. Compulsions can be meaningless—the person trapped into performing them does not have a clear motive or a rationale. For example, counting is a very common compulsion. Some people afflicted with OCD will count every step they take, every mouthful of food they eat, even every Fruit Loop in their bowl of cereal. Sometimes the counting can be an attempt to distract the mind with a task, in order to keep painful obsessive anxieties at bay.

The most common anxieties behind obsessions and compulsions are fears of being contaminated, of failing to perform routine tasks and duties, of hurting others, of inappropriate sexual behavior, or of committing a crime. Even though people with OCD might be obsessed with some fantastic worry that they will grab a knife and stab their spouse, they are not violent people and do not harbor any terrible secrets, hatred, or conflicts. OCD sometimes runs in families, perhaps due to inherited biochemical abnormalities.

Superstitious rituals are a form of compulsion—walking backward to undo your mistake if you stepped under a ladder, throwing salt over your shoulder to ward off bad luck, or avoiding black cats. Sounds childish? Exactly! If you remember back to your own childhood or watch your own children, you can see that some degree of obsessive-compulsive behavior is a natural part of growing up. Children have many rituals for protecting themselves from bogeymen and bad luck. Some will develop their own secret chants and prayers to deal with the anxiety of sleeping alone in a dark room. Other rituals are passed on from generation to generation. Do you remember chanting "Step on a crack, break your mother's back"?

For most children, the need for rituals and magic incantations passes with time. For some, perhaps about one in a hundred, the rituals and compulsions will persist and intensify. Some will give up the childhood rituals but develop compulsions later in life, as an adult. About 2 to 3 percent of the population is believed to have OCD.

When does a cautious or fussy habit cross the line and become a problem? Some experts suggest that any obsessive or compulsive ritual that occupies one hour or more a day is OCD that should be treated. Others say, more vaguely but perhaps more helpfully, that obsessions and compulsions are problems when the sufferer and his or her family experience them as problems. Treatment can be behavioral, helping the OCD sufferer gradually taper down the rituals and compulsions. Often, though, this approach is too stressful for the sufferer, since it requires him or her to confront and manage the sometimes severe anxiety hidden beneath the rituals. For this reason, treatment often relies on serotonin-active drugs such as Prozac, Luvox, and Anafranil (clomipramine), another antidepressant shown to be effective for OCD. Traditional talk psychotherapy that attempts to uncover childhood traumas and hidden conflicts is not effective in changing OCD behavior, another indication that the problem is biochemical, not psychological.

What causes OCD? People who suffer from it find that their rituals are effective and essential to calming their underlying anxiety. Based on studies in animals, Princeton researcher Barry Jacobs has suggested that such rituals as hand washing and other repetitive OCD patterns of behavior may be a form of self-medication. In his studies of serotonin activity in cats, he has demonstrated that there is a substantial increase in serotonin system activity while the animal engages in repetitive movements such as chewing, biting, and grooming the fur with the tongue.

If you have any small nervous habits of your own, this may make sense. Why do people bite their nails when stressed? Or pace up and down when they're worried? Do you ever find yourself twisting or worrying a strand of hair or rubbing your face or hands when you're self-conscious? Does chewing gum somehow relax tension for you? Dr. Jacobs also suggests that the serotonin-enhancing effects of repetitive movement can be used to improve depressed or anxious moods, an idea that will be covered in greater detail in chapter 10.

Can't Forget the Horror

"Shell shock" was the term used when post-traumatic stress disorder (PTSD) was first recognized in World War I soldiers. About 30 percent of

Vietnam combat veterans and 8 percent of Gulf War veterans suffered from it. More recently, 9/11 survivors and rescue workers, as well as returning Iraq war veterans, have demonstrated its symptoms. Survivors of rape, other physical assault, serious car accidents, and plane crashes, or fires, floods, earthquakes, and other natural disasters, can all be tormented by PTSD for months, even years, following their trauma. The symptoms of PTSD include insomnia, vivid nightmares, daytime flashbacks, numbing emotional detachment, extreme jumpiness, intense anxiety when associations and memories are triggered, and profound survivor guilt. Compassionate psychotherapy, support groups, and antidepressant treatment can all help alleviate the distress, but some symptoms, such as nightmares, flashbacks, and the anxiety they bring, can persist for years, even decades after the events that caused PTSD.

Good Reasons for Feeling Anxious

Some people are aware that little things are throwing them into a panic, that they are fretting needlessly. On the other hand, many of us simply have a lot to worry about. You may have a high-stress job where you are under constant pressure to perform. Or you might have a small business of your own where you have to watch the cash flow very carefully. Your kids could have serious school and behavior problems that they may or may not grow out of. You or someone you love might have a worrisome chronic illness. Perhaps your parents are getting frail and can't take care of themselves much longer. These kinds of troubles and fears aren't cured by whistling a happy tune.

As a disorder, anxiety is hard to study because it is difficult to separate reasonable concerns from needless worry. For example, various studies have reported very different rates of anxiety in the elderly—quite low or quite high. We know that serotonin levels decline with age, increasing the risk of depression and anxiety. Yet seniors are often dealing with such unfixable problems as the hardships of living on low fixed incomes, reduced physical mobility or multiple chronic diseases, declining memory and concentration, and perhaps living in much less comfortable or safe surroundings. They are also approaching the ultimate anxiety, death. Wouldn't you worry, too?

Doctors often need to decide whether the elderly widow, the too-busy executive, or the patient with multiple sclerosis has a true anxiety disorder, because they may want to suggest medical treatment. When it comes to making stress-reducing and mood-lifting nutritional and lifestyle changes, it doesn't matter whether your anxiety is realistic or unrealistic, healthy or unhealthy. Any natural intervention that can calm an overactivated mood and promote sleep and relaxation will help you two ways—reducing needless worrying and strengthening you to cope more effectively with legitimate problems.

7

Out-of-Control: Overeating, Drinking, Addictions

In the Middle Ages, European peasants told mouthwatering tales of the fabulous land of Cockaigne. In this mythical kingdom, mountains of cheese and meadows of candy flowers surrounded lakes of delicious meat swimming in sauce. The streams flowed with wine, and everyone could eat and drink to his heart's content. For the medieval peasant, always on the verge of starvation, Cockaigne was truly paradise. For us, accustomed to fully stocked refrigerators and fast-food buffets, it is perfectly ordinary.

Millions of Americans are overweight. They diet, lose weight, and gain it back again. Why do we overeat? Most simply, because we can. We are surrounded by an abundance of food—especially highly refined processed food loaded with sugar and fat. Wherever we go, people put food in front of us, and we often eat under stressful or distracting conditions. A departmental meeting is all bad news except for the donuts and cookies. A coworker bakes brownies and insists that you try one. You grab convenience food for lunch and eat it at your desk. Because it's mostly fat and sugar, you are hungry again before the afternoon is over and get a bag of chips from the vending machine, though you swore you wouldn't. You know you ought to do some kind of exercise when you get home,

138

but you really need to relax and unwind in front of the TV. At least the takeout you brought home for dinner *looks* low in calories.

By way of comparison, imagine living on a farm in the early 1900s. All food is prepared from scratch with fresh, homegrown ingredients. There is plenty to eat, with a balanced selection of meat and dairy foods, vegetables, fruits, and grains. Between meals, everyone has field work or other chores to do. There might be some leftover pie or fried chicken in the icebox for eating between meals, but there are no candy bars, chips, fries, or sugary sodas to be had. You are unlikely to become seriously overweight in this plain-eating, hardworking world. You are also much less likely to fall victim to the diseases of civilization that are believed to be promoted by diets high in sugar or animal fat: adult-onset diabetes, breast cancer, prostate cancer, heart disease, and bowel disease, such as rectal cancer and diverticulosis.

Food Is Everywhere, but Only Thin Is Beautiful

An outrageous abundance of food, plus a societal preoccupation with thinness, are the essential preconditions for eating disorders. Cultures where food is less plentiful and plumpness is considered attractive do not have eating disorders.

An eating problem can be formally defined as being 15 to 20 percent below or above normal body weight. But perhaps a better definition is simply a negative, guilty, obsessed, or anxious preoccupation with food and with eating.

How common are eating disorders? Studies suggest that one out of ten college-age women has significant abnormal eating behavior—either binge eating, bulimia, or anorexia. Binge eating is normally defined as eating a very large amount of food within a two-hour period, sometimes a whole day's worth of calories. The binger usually feels out of control, unable to stop the binge until the food is gone. Some people may binge an average of once a week, while others may have daily binge episodes. In bulimia, binge eating is regularly followed by an attempt to rid the body of the excess calories—either by induced vomiting, laxatives, fasting, or excessive exercise. Both bingeing and purging are often done in secret. The individual may eat normal or below-normal amounts of food in social settings. Anorexia, which is a radical reduction in food intake that can be life-threatening, is relatively uncommon.

Adolescent girls and young women are particularly at risk for eating disorders, since they are greatly preoccupied with their changing bodies; are especially sensitive to rejection by peers who judge on appearances; and may base their self-worth largely on their physical attractiveness. Fashion models and other ultrathin celebrities, whose unrealistic and often unnatural proportions are on display at every newsstand, may encourage them to set rigid, impossible-to-attain standards for themselves.

Eating disorders often begin in the teen years, but they do not necessarily go away with greater maturity. They may in fact become worse. Studies show that women who begin as intensive dieters or mild bingers can progress to more severe eating problems, such as anorexia and bulimia. A well-established pattern of bingeing to relieve distress will, quickly or slowly, inevitably lead to being seriously overweight or obese in later years. As many as 23 to 46 percent of people seeking treatment for obesity report having a significant problem with binge eating.

Do You Have an Eating Disorder?

An estimated 5 million American women do. The following feelings and behaviors are all indicators of a possible eating disorder, either bulimia, binge eating, or anorexia.

- Do you sometimes eat very large amounts of food within a two-hour timeframe, while feeling powerless to stop?
- Do you eat large amounts of food when you are not hungry?

- Do you use forced vomiting, laxatives, or water pills to lose weight?
- Do you overuse or misuse weight-loss products?
- Do you exercise to the point of muscle or joint pain or exhaustion for the purpose of controlling your weight?
- Do you skip two meals or more a day or cut your calorie intake below 500 to control your weight?
- Do you think obsessively about food much of the time? Do you feel that food controls your life?
- Do you lie about binge eating or hide your eating and your food supplies from others?
- Do you feel anxious or irritable if you are somewhere where you can't easily obtain food?
- Do you ever steal food?
- Do you feel disgusted with yourself, depressed, or guilty after bingeing or overeating?
- Do you hate your body or obsess about parts of your body you think are too fat?
- Do you base your self-worth largely on your weight or your body size?
- Do you practice extreme calorie restriction diets?
- Is your target weight much lower than the normal weight for your height?

Serotonin, Appetite, and Impulse

The sight and smell of tempting food, the memory of the pleasure of eating, and the pangs in the stomach would seem to be the key signals telling us it's time to eat. We might not eat at all, however, if it were not for the chemical signals in the tiny portion of the brain called the hypothalamus. The activity of the hypothalamus not only rings the dinner bell in our brains; just as importantly, it tells us when we have had enough.

The eating behavior of animals can be drastically changed by destroying tiny groups of cells in the hypothalamus. Damage to one area of the hypothalamus will cause an animal to refuse food and water altogether, while damage to another will cause an animal to eat to the point of bursting. No direct comparison to human behavior can be made, but it is certainly possible that extremes of overeating and self-starvation may be due to malfunctioning of the hypothalamic appetite-control center.

Changing serotonin levels in the hypothalamus will also change eating behavior, as explained in chapter 2. Decreasing serotonin availability to the hypothalamus will increase food intake, and increasing serotonin availability will decrease food intake. The differences in feeding behavior are substantial.

Although other brain chemicals also affect appetite and eating behavior, serotonin appears to be responsible for overseeing the process. Its influence on motivating "needed" food intake is still not clear; other brain chemicals (such as neuropeptide Y) may be more important for stimulating hunger and appetite. *However, serotonin appears to have a crucial role in inhibiting excessive food intake.* In an important review of serotonin and appetite, University of Leeds researcher John Blundell concluded that serotonin may be the body and brain's means for monitoring every stage of food intake and digestion. The digestive tract, in fact, is plentifully supplied with serotonin receptors that are believed to help gage our nutritional needs and their fulfillment.

We crave and consume more than just meat, potatoes, and donuts, of course. Research with both humans and animals suggests that serotonin has a role in moderating or controlling all our drives to consume substances—food, water, alcohol, and addictive substances ranging from cigarettes to heroin. Yet more broadly, there is tantalizing evidence to suggest that serotonin has pervasive effects on controlling appetites and impulses. Treating animals with serotonin-lowering drugs or diets (as in the tryptophan depletion experiment) will unleash a spectrum of normally inhibited behaviors—increased eating, sexual activity, and aggressiveness. In clinical studies, people with problems related to impulse control, such as addictions, sexual misconduct, or aggression, will have signs of reduced serotonin system activity when compared to healthy volunteers. There is even a well-established link between low serotonin activity and compulsive gambling.

It would be much too simple to equate serotonin with will power, and an insult to the complexity of human nature. Yet the brain can't think and the body can't move without the combined activity of dozens of neurotransmitters. If serotonin activity is reduced for some reason, we are not compelled to behave in any particular way. In fact, lowered or otherwise abnormal serotonin activity can produce opposite effects in different individuals. Some people will overeat when their mood is down, while others will lose their appetites. Some will sleep too much and others too little. We can master our moods and impulses, and regularly do, by giving our attention to some distracting or invigorating activity. Yet it seems clear that reduced serotonin system functioning will reduce our capacity to control our appetites and impulses.

To date, there is no serotonin-active drug that reliably treats binge eating and other impulse control problems. Prozac often, but not always, suppresses appetite and yields a modest weight loss of a few pounds. It can also reduce the number of episodes of binge eating for compulsive overeaters. A few people will gain weight while taking Prozac, perhaps because their appetite was poor while they were depressed.

There is unlikely to be a miracle drug for treating overeating or alcoholism any time soon. For one thing, all our available drugs interact with multiple serotonin receptors throughout the brain and body, so that they can have many undesirable side effects. In this context, the most infamous example of undesirable side effects came with the very popular weight-loss treatment Fen-Phen. Pondimin, or fenfluramine (the Fen of Fen-Phen), and the related drug dexfenfluramine (Redux, basically an "extra strength" formulation of fenfluramine) were marketed as treatments for obesity but widely prescribed to people who just wanted to lose a few pounds. Both drugs were withdrawn from the market in 1997 after studies showed that almost one-third of the patients treated with Fen-Phen had abnormal echocardiograms, suggesting heart valve damage from the drugs. In fact, there had been indicators of potentially dangerous side effects (discussed in the 1996 edition of this book) before Redux was ever approved, but the drug was virtually guaranteed approval in a nation in which one-third of the population is now classified as obese. Both Pondimin and Redux acted to suppress appetite by increasing serotonin availability in the brain, particularly the hypothalamus, creating a sense of fullness and curbing the desire to eat. Other serotonin-active antiobesity drugs are now in development.

Safety concerns regarding antiobesity drugs are not limited to Redux and Pondimin. A recent review by Canadian researchers (published in the January 6, 2007, issue of *The Lancet*), concluded that the studies of current and investigational weight loss drugs have been inadequate to determine their long-term safety and efficacy. The drugs discussed are Xenical (orlistat) and Meridia (sibutramine), plus a third drug, Acomplia (rimonabant), that has not yet received FDA approval. Like Redux, these drugs are only modestly effective, producing an average weight loss of eight or ten pounds. None of these three drugs has been subjected to long-term testing.

At least for the antidepressants, which can be prescribed for obesity accompanied by mood disorders, there are more long-term safety data. Although antidepressant drug therapy may raise mood and occasionally have some modest weight-loss benefit, it will not change ingrained behavior patterns, such as overeating when stressed. Prozac has FDA approval as a treatment for bulimia, but the success rates are in fact very low, with some studies showing no advantage over placebo. A 2005 study found that Prozac was a less effective treatment for binge eating than cognitive behavioral therapy, which helps change basic eating behavior, such as psychological dependence on food for comfort or to lessen anxiety or tension. In the absence of a cure, choosing foods and activities that will enhance serotonin system functioning is a rational and healthy approach to improving appetite and impulse control.

Carb-Craving Binges

Bingeing occurs most often during winter blues or in response to stress and low mood or the hormonal fluctuations of PMS. Almost everyone has had the unhappy experience of compulsively eating a food that they are not really enjoying—eating without real appetite, without really tasting, not stopping until the bag or the carton or the plate is empty. While we binge, we are almost in a trance. The effect is calming, even sedating. We may be ashamed of how much we ate and guiltily hide the empty bag or container, but the tension, anger, anxiety, boredom, or loneliness that impelled us to binge is magically gone, at least for a while.

The drive to eat in response to a disappointment, frustration, or setback isn't hard to understand. Food soothes the stressed adult just as surely as it does a crying baby. Some people will seek out particular foods to ease their feelings. You can probably make out your own list of favorites, but certain categories of foods tend to be selected over and over again by both occasional and chronic bingers as their comfort foods:

- ice cream, pudding, milk
- cookies, cakes, donuts, pastries
- crackers, muffins, bread, cereal
- candy, chocolate
- peanut butter
- pizza
- macaroni-and-cheese
- chips, pretzels, popcorn

It has often been noticed that many people regularly select carbohydrates as their binge or comfort foods. To a certain extent, this is because carbohydrate snacks are the most readily available. Vending machines offer mostly carbo snacks, and every convenience store provides a varied selection placed near the register for impulse purchases. The fact that many of these foods are also high in fat or added sugar makes them more appealing. Although many people prefer the high-calorie hit of cookies or chips, others will binge on straight carbohydrates like crackers. At mealtime, they will tend to have multiple servings of pasta or potatoes rather than meat or fish. In short, carbohydrates seemed to be preferred for reasons that go beyond fat, sugar, and other taste preferences, suggesting the binger may have a metabolic need that the carbohydrates satisfy.

A number of researchers have argued that carbohydrate craving and bingeing may be a direct response to low serotonin system functioning. A carbohydrate meal does increase the brain's supply of tryptophan, allowing more serotonin to be produced and released. In other words, craving carbohydrates during PMS, SAD, or anxiety-provoked bingeing may be a way of self-medicating a serotonin deficiency. Animals who are serotonin-deficient will also tend to select carbohydrates in preference to protein. Craving carbohydrates may not be a taste preference but rather an attempt to restore chemical balance to the brain and body. If this is so, and considerable research does support it, careful selection and timing of carbohydrate intake can improve mood and eliminate the cravings that provoke an out-of-control binge.

The serotonin hypothesis of carbohydrate craving is still controversial, with different groups of researchers reporting very different findings. Those skeptical argue that the protein content of most normal meals is too high to trigger a difference, although other groups of researchers do find an increased proportion of tryptophan in the blood after a mostly carbohydrate meal. As for measuring mood effects of different meal compositions, this is done under (necessarily) such artificial conditions that any mood differences might have been lost.

For example, in one such experiment, female college students were given a meal that was either high protein (6 ounces chicken breast plus 1 tablespoon of Italian dressing, accompanied by 2 ounces of mozzarella plus three saltines) or high carb (white rice with 1 tablespoon of margarine). Over the course of the next three hours, they had to undergo five blood draws and a battery of psychological tests, in between watching an educational documentary. Both groups had roughly equivalent declines in mood, but wouldn't you, too, under such conditions? If you found out that, in exchange for a free lunch of white rice with margarine and a bit of pocket money, you had to undergo five blood draws, plus a lot of tests, and (for entertainment) watch a documentary about rain forests, would you be excited? It is true that valid scientific experiments need to be done under rigidly controlled, uniform conditions, but in this instance the conditions may have been too uniformly depressing to tell us much about the effects of carbohydrates versus protein on mood. Other studies conducted under more lifelike conditions have found that depressed women (including those with PMS or SAD) do seem to have enhanced mood after carbohydrate meals, while other researchers have reported that carbohydrate meals are sedating for people who have no mood problems.

A study performed by Walter Kaye and colleagues at the University of Pittsburgh examined the mood-and-food effects of the now-classic tryptophan depletion experiment on bulimic women. The women with bulimia increased their calorie intake and showed a marked lowering in mood in response to the reduction in brain tryptophan supply and serotonin production. The effects were significantly greater than they were for a comparison group of nonbulimic women who also participated in the experiment. The researchers concluded that bulimics may be much more vulnerable to the effects of temporary shifts in tryptophan availability. Potentially, binges could be triggered by insufficient dietary tryptophan, and a carbohydrate binge could improve mood and appetite control, at least temporarily.

Some people can binge under stress and still keep a normal body weight, though they may "feel fat" and ashamed because of their bingeing. Often, though, bingeing adds pounds that cannot be easily shed. Too many fad diets claim you can shed pounds by avoiding so-called fattening carbohydrates. The stress and deprivation of dieting, particularly low-carbohydrate dieting, will invariably trigger a binge. Irregular meals and inadequate nutrition can also create a hidden agenda for bingeing. *In fact, low-calorie diets reduce blood tryptophan levels, producing a drop in brain serotonin levels.* Howard Steiger, professor of psychiatry at McGill University, and director of an eating disorders program, has proposed that some people with bulimia and impulse control problems have a baseline low serotonin system functioning that can be worsened by dieting, making them more prone to impulsivity or bingeing or both.

This is also the view of Oxford researcher Philip Cowen and colleagues, who have done a series of studies of the effects of restrictive dieting in women with mood or eating disorders. *They have reported that, even in healthy symptom-free women, moderate dieting for three weeks lowered blood levels of tryptophan and impaired brain serotonin system functioning.* When women with a history of bulimia undergo the tryptophan depletion experiment, they experience a return of their mood symptoms and their food obsessions. They conclude that dieting decreases tryptophan availability to the brain, which may in turn trigger the development of bulimia nervosa in susceptible women.

In a society where people binge-eat because they're stressed or depressed, then go on a diet to fix the damage or punish themselves, the impact of dieting on serotonin is an important issue that will be discussed in more detail in part three. The overall best approach to keeping food cravings under control is by choosing healthy, balanced carbohydrates on a schedule that anticipates your daily, monthly, and seasonal mood shifts.

When Bingeing Becomes Routine: Compulsive Overeating

People who binge on a daily basis are often very aware of how their eating is triggered by pent-up negative moods and feelings. They will say they "stuff down" their feelings—get them under control—by stuffing the food into their mouths. Often they are women who have been taught that being pretty and sweet are the secrets to success, and the only qualities that others would value in them. They may have grown up in families where feelings were rarely expressed and they may not feel entitled to display negative feelings such as anger or resentment. Chewing and devouring food becomes a way to express anger, but ultimately the sufferers direct their negative feelings inward, hating their bodies and themselves for being unable to master the compulsion to eat.

For people truly troubled by compulsive overeating, the impulse does not stop with a single bag of chips. They will eat well beyond feeling hunger, even continuing when their jaws and stomachs ache, until the feeling of calm and sedation allows them to stop. Often they then try to discipline themselves, or fix the damage, by dieting. But dieting will bring on feelings of frustration and deprivation, which can only be escaped by another reckless plunge into pizza or cookies or ice cream. Dieting also potentially increases nutritional imbalances that result in lower serotonin availability, as we'll see below.

Chronic binge eating (binge eating disorder) has only recently been recognized as an eating disorder and has not yet been thoroughly studied. Some estimates put the number of binge eaters at 5 million adult Americans, about 60 percent of them women. Major life stresses, chronic depression, traumatic events, and childhood or adolescent sexual abuse are all risk factors for binge eating disorder.

Bulimia: The Cycle of Bingeing and Purging

We reach for a bag of chips, a half gallon of ice cream, intending to have just a taste. To our horror and self-disgust, we finish the whole thing. We feel as though we have suddenly become grotesquely fat. In bulimia, this feeling is so intolerable that the individual must make amends by purging the body of the excess—either by forced vomiting or large doses of laxatives—or by frantic exercising.

Bulimics are not easily pigeonholed or categorized. Some are normal weight, while others are overweight or obese. Some are obsessive, self-controlled, and perfectionistic, while others are just the opposite. Many have other problems with impulse control or addiction, such as alcoholism or compulsive shopping and resulting credit card debt. Some become bulimic in response to repeated, unsuccessful attempts to diet. The deprivation and discomfort of the diet will trigger a binge, which will be followed by purging or stringent dieting, until an overwhelming sense of deprivation brings on another binge. Bulimics are often secretive about their behavior and hide their binges and purges from others. Their repeated cycles of bingeing and purging (or fasting) can take a significant toll on their health. They may have hidden nutritional deficiencies despite maintaining normal or above-normal weight.

Studies have shown that bulimic patients have below-normal serotonin system activity. It is not clear whether their low serotonin activity is the cause or the result of their bulimia. Low serotonin functioning could be related to emotional distress or abnormal appetite and impulse control, which could result in bulimia. Or nutritional deficiencies caused by bulimia could lower the brain's serotonin production, which might make the mood and food cravings still worse. Professor Howard Steiger has proposed that the binge phase of the diet-and-binge cycle may be chemically triggered by a reduction in brain serotonin levels that occurs on a strict low-calorie diet—a theory that will be discussed in greater detail in part three.

Body-Image Distortions

A negative obsession with food almost always includes an obsession, usually an unhappy one, with body image. According to a Harris poll, three-quarters of women and more than half of men say they are dissatisfied with their bodies. Among women, 78 percent are unhappy with their weight and 35 percent would like to lose 25 pounds or more. A concern with our bodies and our physical attractiveness can promote better nutrition, exercise, and self-care. All too often, though, it becomes an obsession that fuels self-loathing and unhealthy eating behaviors—either severe dieting or cycles of bingeing and purging. Bulimics are especially prone to hate their bodies and feeling uncomfortable and alienated from their own physical selves. The more they lose control over their eating behavior, the more they may see themselves as trapped within a huge body with a devouring mouth.

In many cases, these body images are quite distorted. We all know someone who has lost weight to the point of being perhaps too thin, but who still insists on losing more. Many women of normal or near-normal weight are convinced that their thighs or buttocks are disgustingly fat. They may diet strenuously, attempting to make a normal-sized body resemble the unrealistic proportions of a supermodel. A few French fries or one unauthorized dessert will bring on guilt, loathing, and acts of self-punishment and deprivation. Their efforts to lose weight and to change their natural body proportions can lead to nutritional deficiencies that may include reduced serotonin functioning.

Ninety to 95 percent of sufferers from eating disorders—bulimia, bingeing, or anorexia—are female. Is this overwhelming gender difference cultural or chemical? Is it because our culture makes thinness the standard for feminine beauty and popularity, or do women have a chemical and hormonal susceptibility to eating disorders? Both may contribute. As explained in chapter 2, women have lower rates of brain serotonin synthesis compared to men. This biological difference leaves women more susceptible to stress-linked reductions in serotonin levels, which affect appetite and impulse. Interestingly, severe body-image distortions have been linked with serotonin abnormalities and successfully treated with serotonin-active medication.

The most extreme body-image distortions are those of anorexics, who will starve themselves to skeletal thinness yet still insist that they are fat, that their bodies are huge and disgusting. Anorexia is difficult to cure and can be fatal. Between 5 and 20 percent of anorexics will die from the disorder, usually from a combination of heart failure and imbalances of potassium, chloride, and other electrolytes. Anorectic sufferers will sometimes deny symptoms and fight attempts to provide emergency intravenous feedings.

Anorexia, the Ultimate in Self-Control

Self-starvation—anorexia nervosa—occurs in 1 to 5 percent of the population, mostly white adolescent girls and young women. Less severe forms of fasting and extreme dieting are probably much more common. Anorexia can begin when an overweight girl or woman begins a diet that goes out of control. Some will eat and purge, others will consistently restrict food intake to 500 calories a day or less. Apparently, starvation can cause the release of the body's natural opium-like chemicals, the endorphins, so the individual can become addicted to the high of fasting. Despite their fragile, skeletal appearance, anorexics are often highly athletic, exercising strenuously and compulsively even very late in the course of their starvation, perhaps to further stimulate the release of endorphins. In one report, ReVia (naltrexone), a drug used to treat heroin and other substance abuse, was used successfully to treat anorexia, suggesting that self-starvation does produce an addictive high.

Anorexic patients show signs of abnormal serotonin system functioning. While they are actively anorectic and underweight, they appear to have abnormally low serotonin activity, possibly because their extremely low calorie intake has made them deficient in dietary tryptophan. When their weight is restored to normal or near normal, anorectic patients are reported to have abnormally high serotonin activity. People with anorexia tend to be perfectionistic, rigid, and inhibited. Dr. Walter Kaye and colleagues at the University of Pittsburgh have suggested that these people might suffer from a hyperactive serotonin system that predisposes them to be so extremely self-controlled that they can fast to the point of starvation and exercise to exhaustion. They may also have a reduced drive to eat and feel full after eating just a little because of their increased serotonin activity. Their self-starving may be a response to serotonin hyperactivity that acts to adjust serotonin functioning downward by reducing the brain's supply of tryptophan. In fact, anorexic patients report that restricting food intake does make them feel better.

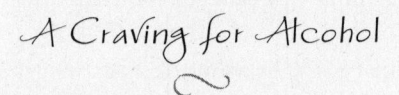

A Craving for Alcohol

Humans are not the only creatures to enjoy alcohol, just the only ones who know how to manufacture it. Birds will gorge themselves silly on fermented fruits and berries, and laboratory mice and rats are readily hooked on alcohol and drugs, making them good models for studying and treating substance abuse in humans. Some of these animal studies have produced fascinating results. For instance:

- Animals that have been stressed will choose alcohol in preference to water to a marked degree.
- Animals kept in darkness will drink more alcohol.
- Treatments that increase brain serotonin levels will reduce alcohol consumption.
- Treatments that reduce brain serotonin levels will increase alcohol consumption.

Many humans are all too aware of how alcohol becomes overwhelmingly attractive in times of stress or anxiety. Some people respond to the depression and craving brought on by SAD by drinking heavily during the winter. It appears as though the serotonin abnormalities that lead to overeating in some people result in excessive alcohol consumption in others. As serotonin-related conditions, alcoholism, depression, and eating disorders are closely linked.

There is a fairly clear link between lowered serotonin functioning and increased drinking. Abnormal serotonin activity can result in feelings of depression and anxiety, creating a motive to seek alcohol. More fundamentally, lowered serotonin activity has what researchers call a "permissive effect" on alcohol drinking, as it does on eating. Appetites and cravings are stimulated, while impulse control, the power to control the craving, is reduced. Incidentally, heavy drinking and impulsive eating problems often coexist. Estimates are that about one-quarter to

153

one-half of those who seek treatment for bulimia will also have an alcohol problem.

It is thought that many heavy drinkers crave alcohol as a treatment for their underlying depression and anxiety. People who drink more heavily when stressed can understand the impulse to drown their sorrows in alcohol. Most are also aware that while one or two drinks can take the edge off their anxiety or aggravation, continued drinking will depress their mood even further. Although many people use a nightcap to help them sleep, alcohol tends to suppress REM sleep, an important portion of the sleep cycle. You may fall asleep quickly, but wake up several hours later and find it difficult to fall back to sleep.

Alcohol generally depresses coordination or motor control, suppresses pain awareness, sedates or tranquilizes, alters mood, and loosens inhibitions. Alcohol undoubtedly acts on the nervous system in many different ways, yet it seems to exert its effects primarily on behaviors that are regulated by the serotonin system. It appears that alcohol does affect serotonin functioning in ways that match alcohol-induced mood changes—an initial upswing is followed by a decline. A number of animal studies suggest that although an initial dose of alcohol may stimulate serotonin activity, chronic or continued drinking impairs it, perhaps promoting further alcohol intake. Serotonin activity will also drop when chronic drinking is stopped—another reason, perhaps, for the craving that makes quitting so stressful and difficult.

Serotonin-enhancing treatments will decrease alcohol consumption in laboratory animals by as much as 50 percent. Their effects on drinking behavior in humans is much more variable. Since alcohol is an addictive drug, changing any underlying serotonin abnormalities will not undo the addiction, though it may enhance an individual's ability to withstand the craving. For people who drink more heavily in winter or in times of anxiety or stress, but who are not alcohol abusers, medication or lifestyle changes to improve serotonin system functioning can help cut down on drinking.

Serotonin-Deficient, Impulsive, Addicted

~

Bingeing can be provoked by drinking, when our inhibitions are relaxed. How many of us have gobbled down too many appetizers at a party, but felt helpless to stop? Impulsive behaviors of all sorts—from fighting to overeating to drug abuse—appear to be released or promoted when serotonin functioning is low. Risk-taking and reckless behavior of various sorts are also related to low serotonin functioning, and frequently fueled by alcohol or drug abuse.

Addiction may seem like something that happens other places—in back rooms, alleyways or wild, glitzy parties. Yet millions of people are addicted to nicotine or to caffeine. You may well know what it feels like to miss your morning jolt of caffeine—drowsiness, irritability, and perhaps a splitting headache will be your punishment. If you are a heavy coffee drinker, you may find that coffee has lost its capacity to perk your mood and alertness, but you keep on drinking cup after cup because you feel awful without it. That is the nasty reality of an addiction. You start using a substance for its mood- and energy-enhancing effects, but you continue to use it because your mood and energy will go drastically lower without it. What was once done for the sake of a reward is now continued to avoid a punishment.

Many people who are bulimic or binge eaters will readily identify themselves as food addicts, and Overeaters Anonymous takes a twelve-step approach to managing overeating as an addiction. In fact, a recent study in the *Proceedings of the National Academy of Sciences* found that obese patients have activity patterns in the hippocampus and other brain regions that are very similar to those seen in drug addicts. Much like a drug or alcohol addict, bulimics will lie about their habit, hide it from others, and think obsessively about their abused substance, in this case food. They derive little or no pleasure from their binges, but instead feel themselves to be victims of a compulsion. An impulse takes over which they are helpless to resist. Some bingers view themselves as two separate persons—their normal self, and a secret binger who takes over their personality in moments of stress. A few people have been known, in fact, to binge while sleepwalking, making themselves Dagwood sandwiches out of random kitchen ingredients, even pet food or soap.

Sufferers from bulimia often have other forms of poor impulse control. They are at great risk of alcohol or drug abuse. They may drastically overuse diet pills, laxatives, and diuretics (water pills). Though these are not physically addictive, they may go on to abuse amphetamines for their weight-reducing properties. Bulimics may also engage in compulsive shopping or even shoplifting, stealing trivial items that they could easily afford to buy. Impulsive and addictive behaviors, like overeating, can have a sedating and intoxicating effect that relieves anxiety or distress. Like bingeing, compulsive shoplifting is often done in a trance-like state, and the person may not be fully conscious of the act of stealing.

The neurotransmitter dopamine is thought to have a major role in addictions and generally in pleasure-seeking and pain-avoiding behavior. Serotonin appears to act as a brake on the dopamine system, moderating reward- and punishment-driven impulses. A healthy serotonin system helps to withstand overeating and drinking impulses, and to moderate our drives for food, alcohol, sex, and other pleasures. In some instances, as mentioned in chapter 6, serotonin activity may inhibit impulses by causing a mild state of anxiety, enough to make us hesitate before pursuing an attractive but unwise course of action.

Everyday Impulse Problems

Take the common experience of opening a bag of chips or cookies when you're bored or down. You are not really hungry. You only intend to have a couple. Yet you finish the entire bag, not really enjoying it, but unable to marshal the self-control to put it down. Are there other areas of your life where you have similar impulse control problems—other time-, health-, or money-wasting activities that provide more guilt than pleasure, yet are so hard to give up?

Do you shop when you are depressed or discouraged, trying to cheer yourself up with a new wardrobe, home furnishings, or toys? Do you buy yourself gifts for Christmas or Hanukkah when you meant to shop for friends and family? Binge shopping affects an estimated 1 to 6 percent of the population. The typical shopaholic is a woman in her thirties. People who spend from boredom or anxiety are often self-employed or working on a part-time or on-call basis, work situations that create boredom and anxiety. They may also shop as a way of seeking social interactions and enjoying the attentions of the sales clerk. More affluent types may shop online or by catalog for the sake of the brief pleasure of finding a package outside their door when they come home to a dark apartment after a long and dispiriting day of work. Compulsive buying accounts for billions of dollars in credit-card debt. Similar to overeating, an immense variety and abundance of goods, plus universal availability, easy credit, and other buy-now incentives, can spur out-of-control consumption.

More serious impulse control problems include compulsive sexual activities—entering multiple relationships and entanglements that are pursued for the sake of conquest, or for the sake of being valued as a conquest, in either case to prop up one's self-esteem. Many women, in particular, treasure the illusion of being cared for that physical touching and caresses give them. Like any other addiction, the pain of deprivation, of not having a lover, may be the real motive for the sexual activity, rather than the actual pleasure of the moment.

As legalized gambling becomes more common and more readily available, more people have mild to severe problems with controlling their desire to hit it big. A few dollars a day on lottery tickets may or may not have an impact on one's budget, but a weekend trip to a casino certainly can. True compulsive gambling—spending everything one has—is relatively rare. Yet many people will spend hundreds or even thousands of dollars on slot machines and games of chance that they have little likelihood of winning. A small win every now and then feeds the addiction. Even after losing over and over again, it is so much harder to walk away than to put another quarter in the slot. Adolescent addiction to computer games, which can interfere quite substantially with schoolwork, is a similar impulse-control problem.

The rise of the Internet and its many irresistible attractions has produced a range of compulsive and addictive behaviors that are still not well studied. We have all spent an unplanned hour or two at the computer, following link after link of arcane material—an admittedly sedentary activity that can be educational as well as recreational. But some people have a real addiction, spending most of their free time in front of the screen. Sometimes the computer is a private outlet for addictive or compulsive behaviors that might be more embarrassing, expensive, or inconvenient to pursue in the real world, such as sexual obsessions, pornographic interests, or gambling. Simply because the computer is always there and always turned on, impulses to shop, gamble, or both at once (eBay!) are much, much harder to resist. For someone with a shopping, gaming, or gambling habit, a computer is like a kitchen perpetually stocked with chips, cookies, and ice cream.

The analogy is apt because these impulse control problems often coincide. The same individual has issues with binge-eating, drinking, and out-of-control spending. No one has yet done a tryptophan depletion experiment with compulsive buyers or gamblers. (What would that involve? Giving them a wad of cash and then dropping them off at the mall or the track?) But there is a very substantial body of evidence to say that all these impulse control problems—bingeing, overeating, drinking, overspending, and gambling—are linked to low serotonin levels or reduced serotonin system activity.

Seriously Out-of-Control

Everyone has seen the drunk who gets out of hand—arguing, picking fights, becoming verbally or physically abusive. Domestic violence is very often triggered by alcohol, when it lowers normal impulse control and allows repressed anger and aggression to rage uncontrolled. Only certain people are prone to becoming a mean drunk when intoxicated. Others get giggly, flirtatious, boastful, self-pitying, or just sleepy. The link that binds aggression and alcohol consumption appears to be serotonin system deficiencies.

In animals there is a clear correlation between violence and low serotonin levels. Diets and drug treatments that decrease brain serotonin levels will reliably result in increased aggression in rats, mice, and monkeys. Tame animals, such as laboratory rats, tend to have higher serotonin activity than their wilder and more aggressive counterparts.

As a modulator or inhibitor of impulsive and aggressive behavior, serotonin basically helps us get along with others. Self-control, empathy, and cooperation are complex, *learned* social skills. All the same, people who are unable to master these fundamental social behaviors may have serotonin system deficiencies. Many studies have found markers of reduced serotonin activity in adults with a history of aggression or poor impulse control, ranging from compulsive gambling and addiction to explosive rage and repeated violent crimes. Children who are highly aggressive or extremely cruel to animals, or who set fires or commit significant acts of vandalism, have been shown to have signs of reduced serotonin activity. Children with these types of impulse and conduct disorders do not necessarily go on to commit crimes as adults; however, they are at high risk of becoming alcoholic or addicted.

We tend to think of suicide as the act of someone severely depressed or despairing, perhaps because of some major loss, like the death of a spouse. In fact, suicide can be an act of impulse on the part of someone who may have suffered a sudden stress, such as the breakup of a relationship. If the attempt is unsuccessful, the individual may not really know why he or she did it, and may have made the attempt in an almost trance-like state. Depression, alcohol, and poor impulse control can collude in causing acts of violence against others or oneself. Clinical studies of suicide attempters and autopsies of suicide victims have shown significantly diminished serotonin functioning. Some of these very unfortunate people were not terribly unhappy or severely depressed, and their act of self-destruction may have been impulsive, sudden, and unplanned. Often their friends and families suffer unnecessarily by thinking that they failed them somehow, when not even hindsight and bitter grief can find a reason for the suicide.

Putting It All Together

Someone who is merely troubled by moodiness and an inability to put down a bag of potato chips before it is empty may be alarmed or even offended by discussions of violence, suicide, and addiction. People with mild mood and food problems should *not* see themselves as ill or at risk for these severe psychiatric disorders. Nor is it implied that the serotonin system *by itself* determines whether someone is depressed, bulimic, or addicted—or merely moody and prone to headaches.

The serotonin theory simply proposes that this neurotransmitter plays a major role in controlling and adjusting mood, appetite, impulse, and pain awareness. Serotonin activity normally fluctuates with the time of day and season of year, and in women with the time of month. Events in our lives, stresses such as an illness or a personal loss or disappointment, can also cause serotonin function to fluctuate or to drop. Some people have an innate serotonin system deficiency or instability that makes them more vulnerable to environmental factors and to stress. Any inherited serotonin deficiencies may well be aggravated by the fact that we are all out-of-sync with the natural world. Our schedules are disconnected from the day-night cycle, our jobs are mostly sedentary, and we have given up traditional eating habits that rely on complex carbohydrates (whole grains, fruits, and vegetables) as staples.

An inherited serotonin system instability can be expressed in any of a myriad different behaviors and responses. A highly dysfunctional or abusive family and a stressful environment might make someone more prone to aggression or addiction. Good circumstances and generally good genes might keep the mood and impulse problems to a minimum. Depending on the dice life rolls you—on your upbringing, environment, and life history—you might be inclined to mood swings, winter blues, and binge eating. Someone else in these circumstances might be anxious and obsessive or prone to insomnia or to migraine.

None of these tendencies are irreversible or unavoidable. You can take control by changing some of the dietary and environmental factors that promote serotonin fluctuations. Cognitive behavior therapy or medication must be the treatment of choice for persons suffering from real impairment in their ability to function and to enjoy life. People who are having acute problems with mood or eating because of a major life stress might also benefit from therapy or a short course of antidepressants. For others, the eating and activity program outlined in the following chapters will provide good to excellent control over symptoms, along with the satisfaction of doing it yourself through a side-effect-free healthy lifestyle.

Part Three

~

Boosting Serotonin Naturally

8

Does "Food and Mood" Equal "Food and Serotonin"?

The food-mood connection is one that most, perhaps all, people have experienced. It has been the subject of relatively little research, perhaps because of the difficulty of documenting subtle shifts in behavior achieved through food, compared to those that are the results of treatment with powerful drugs. The little research that has been done on this major topic suggests that serotonin may be a major component in the mood-elevating response to eating. In fact, to date, it is the only mood-food link for which there is extensive scientific data.

Whether a newborn baby or the CEO of a company, people tend to become irritable or depressed when they are hungry and experience at least a momentary mood lift when they satisfy that hunger with any available and acceptable food. These mood changes could be relatively straightforward. Low blood sugar makes us irritable or physically and mentally depressed. Eating results in a release of serotonin and possibly endorphins as well, both of which are mood-calming and pain-relieving neurotransmitters. Serotonin release in the hypothalamus may trigger both the feeling of fullness and satisfaction and the improved mood experienced with it.

For decades, many investigators and physicians were skeptical about the mood-altering effects of foods (not counting caffeine, nicotine, and alcohol, which are drugs rather than foods). It was believed that the brain was protected from contamination and somewhat isolated from the body by the so-called blood-brain barrier, which limits the ability of many substances to pass from the bloodstream into the brain. The term blood-brain barrier, as explained in chapter 2, simply means that the blood vessels of the brain are less permeable than the vessels supplying nutrients to the rest of the body. Oxygen and sugar (glucose) reach hungry brain tissues quickly, but large molecules, including the amino acid tryptophan, have a longer, slower passage out of the bloodstream and into the brain.

It was also considered counterintuitive to suppose that an organ so important to survival as the brain could be affected by something so trivial as food choices. While it is true that many substances penetrate the brain only slowly or in limited quantities, much contemporary research suggests the brain does not function in lofty isolation after all. It is part of the endocrine gland system and it is constantly bathed in mood- and thought-altering hormones—as any parent with teenagers or any woman with PMS knows all too well. What's more, brain and belly have much more to do with each other than once supposed. In the course of evolution, the gut came first. It had to do a lot of thinking, feeling, and reacting on its own, long before the brain was a glimmer in the eye of Mother Nature.

Gut Feelings

We often talk about feeling something "on a gut level," perhaps because the digestive tract does seem to register and respond to our emotions. We have butterflies in the stomach or sudden cramping in the gut or feel our throat close up when we feel intense emotions—nervousness, fear, even love. When anxious or depressed, some people will have unexplained gastrointestinal symptoms, such as abdominal pain, chronic diarrhea, or irritable bowel syndrome (covered in greater detail in chapter 5). In the past, it was assumed these problems were all "in the head." Modern, more detailed studies of the anatomy of the nervous system have shown that there is a "second brain" in the gut, which includes a whopping 100 million neurons or nerve cells, more than the spinal cord contains.

This is still a modest number compared to the brain itself, which holds thousands of millions of cells. All the same, the size and complexity of the gut's brain suggests it has important roles to perform. No one has yet suggested that the brain in the gut can think. Yet much evidence suggests that the gut can feel, or at least can influence the feeling and mood states generated in the brain itself. It is largely independent of the brain, unlike the rest of the body's nervous system, but the two nerve centers are also in constant communication. An upset in the brain will trigger a corresponding reaction in the gut, and vice versa, as sufferers from anxiety and gastrointestinal disorders know very well. The importance of the complex nervous system of the gut is just now being appreciated and researched. We may hope to understand more about mood-food and brain-belly connections in the future, such as the explanation for the mysterious fact that constipation can trigger headaches.

This gut-level brain, known as the enteric nervous system, is basically wrapped around the whole gastrointestinal tract, from the throat to the colon. It is just under the lining of the tract, where it can sense and monitor the food and drink being digested. It also has specific sensors for sugar, protein, acidity, and other factors important to digestion. Virtually all the neurotransmitters found in the brain have been found in the gut, including norepinephrine and endorphins, and it is in particular richly supplied with serotonin. In fact, the greatest (by far!) portion of the body's supply of serotonin is found in the enteric nervous system, suggesting it might have an important role for all mood-food links.

Leeds University researcher John Blundell suggests that the regulation of eating may have been one of serotonin's earliest functions. Serotonin evolved long ago in the history of life, and appears to be the first of the neurotransmitters. *Its primitive and still most crucial activities are regulating the two functions most important to the life of an animal—feeding and moving.* It may be the case that serotonin links the brain and belly by signaling the nutritional status and needs of the body. It signals fullness or satiety, and it may also alert the brain to the balance of carbohydrates, fat, and protein in the digestive tract, perhaps influencing food selection for the next meal. It may be the case that gut serotonin is just as significant as brain serotonin in determining how we eat and how we feel. More research is needed.

We are most often aware of how our gut is feeling when it is causing us pain, or reacting to our own negative mood states. It may well be that our mood is being subtly modulated by the gut, and it releases stress or relaxation chemicals in response to the food we eat. If so, food does set our mood, and we truly do feel with our gut.

Food Cravings: Self-Medication or Addiction?

There is a long-lasting controversy over the issue of whether people (and animals) seek and select their foods on the basis of the body's nutritional needs. Animals will go to great lengths to obtain the tiny amounts of salt that are necessary for life, minuscule compared to the amounts human beings liberally shake onto their food. Considering the complex survival traits possessed by both animals and humans, it makes sense to assume that we would have instincts or feedback mechanisms that would direct us to select foods on the basis of our nutritional needs.

Nutritionists who bear witness to the terrible eating habits of Americans have reason to doubt that food cravings and preferences have any nutritional basis. Many obese or overweight Americans may in fact be malnourished in the sense of having subtle vitamin and nutrient deficiencies despite easy access to foods containing the needed nutrients. It appears that both people and some species of animals have a powerful drive for high-fat, high-sugar foods—quick energy foods that would give a survival advantage in an environment where food is relatively scarce and life is hard. Because this drive is so powerful, these foods seem to have a quasi-addictive appeal. In other words, the high-fat, high-sugar preference can overwhelm any instinctive tendency to pick foods based on true nutritional needs.

In fact, research has shown that if you give human beings either pure fat or pure sugar, they will eat only as much as they need to survive. But when fat and sugar are combined in a 40 to 60 percent ratio (as in a fairly standard cake, cookie, or pastry), there is effectively no limit to how much people will eat. As a result, many nutritionists feel it is almost unethical to encourage overfed, yet malnourished Americans to believe that they can rely on their own tastes and preferences to achieve a healthy diet.

There are scientific data supporting the view that food cravings are, at least in part, fueled by nutritional needs. Often, though, the quality of this evidence has been greatly overestimated both by the general public and by scientists, who also like to rationalize their personal food preferences. Some of the wilder and more unsubstantiated claims have been made for chocolate—it's an aphrodisiac, a stimulant!—no, it's a sedative and an antidepressant! Women seem to have especially strong chocolate-seeking drives, particularly during the premenstrual phase. But the craving for rich, luscious chocolate candy and confections transcends gender, age, season, and time. It has been suggested that the chocolate lust might in fact be motivated by a need for the amino acid phenylalanine, which, like tryptophan, is an essential amino acid, one that must be obtained from the diet because it cannot be synthesized by the body. You should not take this dubious and unproven theory as a justification for indulging in chocolates beyond the limits of good health and good sense. We don't have an essential dietary requirement for a food that was only made available to most of the world in the last three hundred years! Some dairy products are much better sources of phenylalanine, yet few people report uncontrollable cravings for cottage cheese. In fact, a recent study found that emotional eaters who chose chocolate as their favorite comfort food actually had a prolonged low mood after indulging themselves, apparently because pleasure was quickly succeeded by guilt. If you eat a lot of chocolate, it is because you like it, not because your body needs it.

A Craving for Bread, or for Cake?

The groundbreaking study on carbohydrates and brain serotonin was published in the journal *Science* in 1972 by MIT researchers John Fernstrom and Richard Wurtman. In it, they established for the first time that the protein and carbohydrate content of a meal can have a powerful impact on the production of this important neurotransmitter. Both have since continued to be leaders in researching the effects of diet on serotonin levels. Though they have presented similar findings on how meals affect mood, they have come to hold very different views on how moods, in turn, affect meals.

Not too surprisingly, the discovery of the importance of serotonin and the effects of carbohydrates on its availability to the brain has occasioned a great deal of speculation and experimentation to determine whether people with low serotonin levels are drawn to carbohydrate foods. In fact, a craving for carbohydrate foods is a prominent feature of both SAD and PMS. About two-thirds of SAD sufferers report increased appetite for carbohydrates during the winter months, with a preference for starches such as pasta, bread, potatoes, rice, and corn. For them these heavy foods brighten mood and reduce fatigue. Their carbohydrate intake will drop during the summer, or during treatment with serotonin-active drugs or L-tryptophan supplements. Similarly, many women will crave carbohydrates in their premenstrual time, and those with significant PMS problems will often show a preference for carbohydrates throughout the month, possibly reflecting an attempt to boost chronically poor serotonin availability. PMS sufferers will also tend to reduce carbohydrate consumption if treated with Prozac or another serotonin-active drug. Finally, many people with bingeing or obesity problems report that they most strongly crave carbohydrates.

Based on their studies of the dietary preferences of people with eating disorders or obesity, researchers Richard and Judith Wurtman have proposed that bingers and overeaters preferentially seek out carbohydrates in an attempt to self-medicate an underlying serotonin deficiency. They propose that there is a sort of feedback loop to regulate serotonin production and carbohydrate consumption. A deterioration in mood or some other serotonin-related symptom will trigger a preference for carbohydrates. Increased carbohydrate consumption will raise brain serotonin levels and temporarily suppress the craving for carbohydrates, while favoring increased intake of protein. This makes such good sense that it seems all but proven, but there are some problems with the "carbohydrate-craving" hypothesis.

Dr. Fernstrom, now at University of Pittsburgh, has continued to research the relationship between serotonin and diet in laboratory animals. He has questioned the carbohydrate-craving theory on a number of grounds. He points out that the studies run by the Wurtmans identify carbohydrate cravers on the basis of their snack selections from a menu of choices in which the carbohydrate snacks are relatively high in fat, sugar, and sex appeal, compared to the protein snacks. Who wouldn't pick Pepperidge Farm granola cookies over Slim Jim beef jerky? In addition, in at least some of these studies, the volunteers were recruited through advertisements looking for self-diagnosed carbohydrate cravers. This suggests that the study participants may not have been blind to the goal of the study.

Dr. Fernstrom also points out, based on studies in animals, that even a small proportion of protein added to a carbohydrate snack may negate its potential to raise brain serotonin. In rats, just 5 percent protein will suppress the meal's ability to affect brain serotonin production. A snack containing nuts, chocolate, or cheese may be mostly carbohydrate, but a preference for such a snack isn't sufficient evidence to support the carbohydrate-craving theory. Many of the meals and snacks preferred by self-proclaimed carbo cravers could have little or no serotonin-related effects on mood.

None of this suggests that carbohydrates do not have the potential to improve mood by raising brain serotonin production. Rather, people who seek chocolaty, buttery, or fried snacks and meals are not necessarily driven by a serotonin-deficient desire for carbohydrates, even though they may be snacking or bingeing because of a serotonin system deficiency. The strong instinctive or cultural preference for fats and sugars might dominate any weaker drive to medicate a serotonin deficit with carbohydrates. If this is so, an individual with a serotonin deficit may tend to select pasta with a cream sauce or creamy chocolate candy as a mood-enhancing or comforting food. Since these foods contain substantial proportions of protein, any improvement in mood or other symptoms may be only momentary, related to the antianxiety effects of all satisfying foods. If it were true that we crave only those foods that satisfy our nutritional needs, two-thirds of all Americans would not be seriously overweight.

Rechanneling this preference for high-fat, high-sugar treats to more wholesome, unprocessed carbohydrates, like whole-grain breads, salads, and fruit, may both improve mood and reduce bingeing. High-fat or high-sugar foods can give a momentary pleasure, often followed by a mood drop and a rapid return of appetite. In contrast, complex carbohydrate foods can provide a sustained mood and energy lift, providing their intake is well timed. Chapter 9 will give guidance on choosing wholesome and appealing feel-good meals and snacks.

The Tryptophan Story

Serotonin is a relatively simple molecule that is produced in the brain and body from the amino acid tryptophan. The enzyme responsible for synthesizing serotonin from tryptophan is "unsaturated" at normal brain levels of tryptophan, simply meaning that under normal conditions the enzyme is not working up to capacity. In fact, it has the potential to produce about ten times as much serotonin as it does under its normal workload. Increasing the supply of tryptophan to the brain will increase serotonin production, and has been shown to do so in numerous experiments with animals.

In studies involving both humans and animals, a tryptophan-deficient diet will trigger depressed mood, irritability, and aggressiveness.

In contrast, administering the dietary supplement L-tryptophan has demonstrated at least some efficacy in relieving depression, migraine, and insomnia. L-tryptophan supplements have also shown value in controlling appetite for people with bulimia or binge eating problems.

"Sound great! Where do I get it?" Well, currently you cannot obtain L-tryptophan supplements in the United States. L-tryptophan had been available as an over-the-counter dietary supplement in the 1980s, when it was used as an "alternative" and sometimes as a "mainstream" treatment for PMS, insomnia, appetite control, pain, anxiety, and depression—all the serotonin-associated conditions. Then, in 1989 and 1990, the sudden occurrence of over 1,500 cases of a rare and potentially fatal condition called eosinophilia myalgia syndrome was traced to L-tryptophan supplements, which were immediately recalled by the FDA. This outbreak of eosinophilia myalgia syndrome was later linked to impurities in one foreign manufacturer's shipment of L-tryptophan. There are still doubts about this product's safety, however, and the FDA has not lifted the ban on L-tryptophan in the United States. It has remained available by prescription in Canada, where there have been no health problems associated with its use.

Another related compound called 5-HTP (5-hydroxytryptophan) is available as an over-the-counter supplement in both the United States and Canada. The commercial product is extracted from the seeds of a West African plant (*Griffonia simplicifolia*). Chemically, the 5-HTP compound is an intermediate between tryptophan and serotonin. In theory, a 5-HTP supplement should be an effective antidepressant, as well as a treatment for other low serotonin conditions. In practice, the oral supplement may have limited influence on mood and behavior if most of the 5-HTP is converted to serotonin in the gut before it has a chance to reach the brain.

Studies comparing 5-HTP to prescription antidepressants or to placebo (a look-alike dummy pill) have reported inconsistent results— some showing the supplement to be as effective as prescription drugs, others showing no advantage over placebo. Many of these studies involved too few patients to produce a statistically convincing result, or were too poorly designed to be entirely trustworthy. The published studies have used doses ranging from 20 to 3,250 mg per day. Lower repeated daily doses (for example, 50 mg three times daily) appear to be more effective with a lower risk of side effects (primarily nausea, vomiting, and diarrhea, probably resulting from increased serotonin production in the gastrointestinal tract). Without careful medical supervision, 5-HTP should not be taken in conjunction with other serotonin-active drugs, such as SSRI antidepressants, because of the risk of serotonin syndrome (as discussed in chapter 2).

With lower doses, 5-HTP supplements would appear to be safe and might well provide excellent symptom control for people who feel more comfortable taking a natural product than a pharmaceutical such as Prozac and Zoloft. Bear in mind, though, that an isolated and purified compound from a seed or a shrub or a flower is no longer natural. We do not find purified, concentrated 5-HTP or L-tryptophan in nature, any more than we can pick Prozac from a tree or dig Zoloft out of the ground. That said, supplements are certainly worth trying, if you do not deceive yourself about their purportedly benign and natural qualities. The problems with the contaminated L-tryptophan supplement, which resulted in thirty-eight deaths, are a grim reminder that there is a tiny but real risk with taking dietary supplements, just as there is with prescription drugs. Low levels of the same impurity were identified in six commercial 5-HTP supplements in a 1998 study by Mayo Clinic researchers. The same group of researchers have also reported related contaminants—again at very low levels—present in melatonin supplements. If you do want to try an over-the-counter melatonin or 5-HTP supplement, look for a brand carrying the ConsumerLab.com (CL) certification seal or the United States Pharmacopia (USP) verification seal.

Whenever you read some promising new health information, whether it is about the latest antioxidant or the newest use for vitamin C, it is best to try to reap the potential benefits from including good natural sources in a well-balanced diet, before trying either supplements or medication. Ultimately, health and well-being don't come in a bottle. Only good lifestyle practices can offer you long-term results that are also free of negative side effects. There are many good food choices that can raise brain tryptophan levels that, fortunately, include many of America's favorite foods.

Tryptophan and Food

Tryptophan is one of the essential amino acids—meaning that the body requires it to make protein but cannot synthesize it from other substances. It must be obtained directly from the diet. As explained in chapter 2, tryptophan is found in all animal protein, including dairy products, meat, and fish. It is also found in nuts, seeds, and some vegetables.

Eating more protein, however, does not boost the brain's production of serotonin. No matter how many cheeseburgers you eat, serotonin production in the brain won't rise above baseline, which is about 10 percent of capacity. This is because of the blood-brain barrier and its specialized transport system, which only allows a limited number of large molecules to pass into the brain at a given time. Smaller nutrients, like sugar molecules, can pass quickly and easily into the brain. The larger amino acid molecules all need to hitch a ride on the specialized amino acid shuttle to pass into the brain—a safety mechanism to keep potentially toxic substances out of the brain. A high-protein meal creates a rush-hour competition for space on the brain-bound protein shuttle. There is only so much room on the shuttle, and tryptophan is one of the less common amino acids, so it easily outnumbered and jostled out of a place on the brain-bound shuttle.

Remember the tryptophan depletion experiment described in chapter 2? After a couple of days of a low-protein diet, drinking a special (very nasty tasting) concoction containing all the normal protein amino acids *except* tryptophan has two immediate results. First, there is suddenly a great deal more competition to board the brain-bound protein shuttle. Second, stimulated by the sudden dose of amino acids after two days of protein deprivation, the body begins to use this opportunity to make more protein, but must use up current stores of tryptophan in order to do so. As a result, almost no tryptophan passes into the brain, and brain serotonin production drops drastically.

Paradoxically, to increase the amount of tryptophan reaching the brain, you have to have a meal or snack consisting almost entirely of carbohydrates—either complex carbohydrates, such as breads, grain, rice, or pasta, or simple carbohydrates, such as table sugar or the sugars found in fruit and vegetables.

How does this work? A carbohydrate meal (or snack) causes the pancreas to release insulin, which regulates the amount of sugar in the bloodstream. One of insulin's many effects is to stimulate muscle tissue to take up specific large amino acids. In effect, insulin operates a muscle-bound protein shuttle that does not accept tryptophan. The competing amino acids hop on board, leaving more room on the brain-bound shuttle for tryptophan, which then begins to pass into the brain in higher concentrations. Tryptophan is present in a great variety of foods, although often at very low levels—1 or 2 percent of total protein. Some researchers have suggested that people with severe eating disorders—anorexia or bulimia with forced vomiting—may have an underlying tryptophan and B vitamin deficiency that results from their chaotic eating habits. However, there is no evidence that people with mild to moderate serotonin-related problems are deficient in dietary tryptophan, and eating more protein— even turkey—will not result in higher tryptophan and serotonin levels.

You have probably heard the popular myth that tryptophan is especially abundant in turkey, and that is why people tend to be sleepy or sedated after Thanksgiving dinner. Actually, according to the USDA's Nutrient Data Laboratory Web site (http://www.ars.usda.gov/ba/bhnrc/ndl), turkey has about the same amount of tryptophan as chicken and a good bit less than roast pork. That familiar postdinner drowsiness is more likely due to overeating. Thanksgiving is the only holiday, after all, that is entirely dedicated to eating! Having just a bite or two of turkey with a large helping of stuffing and cranberry sauce would be the proper recipe for boosting brain serotonin levels.

There are abundant data from animal studies to demonstrate that a carbohydrate meal will increase *both* brain tryptophan *and* brain serotonin levels. It is more difficult to verify that the increase in brain serotonin results in a change in brain functioning. In general, it takes a fairly powerful drug to cause a change in behavior so drastic that it can be measured and quantified. However, the magnitude of the change in serotonin availability after a carbohydrate meal approximates the change observed in the tryptophan depletion studies. The fact that the brain tryptophan supply can be readily altered by food choice does support the theory that a well-timed carbohydrate meal will have a positive impact on mood and other serotonin-related symptoms. A number of studies have been done with human volunteers who are asked to report their mood and energy level after protein or carbohydrate meals. In general, people who have symptoms of serotonin deficiency do report improved mood after carbohydrate consumption.

The Wurtmans and their MIT colleagues performed a small study in 2003 comparing the effects of a high protein versus a high carbohydrate breakfast on tryptophan availability to the brain (estimated by the ratio of tryptophan to the competing amino acids in the bloodstream). The high-carb breakfast consisted of waffles with maple syrup, orange juice, and coffee with sugar. The high-protein breakfast was roughly equivalent to an Egg McMuffin without the muffin. These researchers happily reported a statistically significant difference in tryptophan availability, supporting their previous research on the effects of food on brain serotonin levels. But, quite interestingly, most of the difference resulted from the suppressive effects of the protein breakfast. A high-carb breakfast produced a modest 10 percent increase in tryptophan availability to the brain, whereas the high-protein breakfast knocked baseline tryptophan availability down by 35 percent. Perhaps there is a good biological reason why a woman (who is much more vulnerable to serotonin fluctuations) will so often order a large salad for dinner, while her husband or date has the steak! People who seek carbohydrates during low mood episodes like SAD could be protein avoiding as much as carbohydrate craving.

Timing Is Everything

Experiments with laboratory animals have provided the best data concerning how the timing and the protein and carbohydrate content of meals affect brain serotonin levels. Here's how it works. If the first meal of the day consists mostly of carbohydrates with very little protein, there will be a significant increase in brain serotonin about two to three hours later. If the first meal of the day is mostly protein, no such increase occurs. A combined protein-carbohydrate meal will also produce no change in brain serotonin levels. In other words, if your first meal of the day is the traditional bacon, eggs, and toast, there is too much protein in the meal to increase serotonin production, even though you might experience the mild, momentary mood lift that comes with eating just about anything.

Similarly, consuming carbohydrates relatively soon after a protein or a mixed protein-carbohydrate meal will have little or no effect. All the studies done to date indicate that it takes a low-protein, high-carb snack or meal on an empty stomach to achieve the mood-lifting effects of increased brain serotonin production. In laboratory rats, an interval of three hours seems to be the minimum needed, and it may be somewhat longer for human beings, who have a slower metabolic rate. However, going on the basis of experiments with rats, if the first meal is carbohydrates, the second meal can contain some protein in addition to carbohydrates. The brain levels of tryptophan will remain higher than they would if the first meal contained some protein.

In other words, both when and what you eat are important. Your daily mood and energy fluctuations can be your guide as to how you choose and schedule your meals and snacks. If you tend to be at your worst in the early morning and late afternoon, then you should try a carbohydrate breakfast and have a carbohydrate treat in the late afternoon. But don't eat carbohydrates and nothing but carbohydrates all day in an effort to control your moods. The body's response to each meal, whether protein or carbohydrate rich, will be influenced by the nutritional composition of preceding meals. A carbohydrate meal that follows a protein meal will have a larger effect on boosting brain serotonin levels than a carbohydrate meal following a carbohydrate meal or snack.

Not Just Serotonin: Carbohydrate, Protein, and the Brain

Remember that amino acid shuttle that tryptophan needs to ride in order to cross into the brain? A protein meal results in a rush hour competition for space on that shuttle, so that a huge mob of branched chain amino acids (leucine, isoleucine, and valine) crowd out the aromatic amino acids (tryptophan, tyrosine, and phenylalanine). In contrast, a carbohydrate meal will result in a release of insulin, which triggers a muscle-bound amino acid shuttle that ferries only the branched chain amino acids to the muscles, where they can be used as an energy source. Now more of the aromatic amino acids can pass into the brain.

Tryptophan, as we know, is the precursor or source for making serotonin. Tyrosine (also phenylalanine, which is converted into tyrosine) is the source for two equally important brain chemicals, norepinephrine and dopamine. Like serotonin, these two neurotransmitters have multiple, complex, and often complementary functions in the brain and body. Dopamine is thought to have a major role in pleasure-seeking and pain-avoiding behavioral drives. Norepinephrine is an activating chemical released during stress that, along with serotonin, helps to fine-tune our mood state in response to events around us. Tyrosine and phenylalanine are more abundant in the diet than tryptophan, so the brain's synthesis of dopamine and norepinephrine does not fluctuate as greatly in response to normal mostly protein or mostly carbohydrate meals. However, use of amino acid supplements can have negative effects on the brain's supply of all three neurotransmitters.

Branched chain amino acid (BCAA) supplements have been heavily marketed to athletes, especially bodybuilders. The theory to support their use is a good one, but the real-world evidence that they actually make a difference in athletic performance is not that strong. If you are an athlete who also has serotonin-related issues, such as depression or bulimia, you should avoid BCAA supplements. The evidence for carbohydrate loading as a strategy to improve performance is arguably better than the data to support amino acid supplements. If you are concerned about getting enough protein for muscle development, have a high-protein meal or snack after a workout. Since vigorous exercise almost always raises both mood and serotonin levels, you will likely feel good no matter what you eat.

Give Your Tastes the Mood Test

You will not know whether more carbohydrates (or less protein) can boost your mood until you try, and do so in a fairly scientific way. As a first experiment, try changing the meal or snack you consume at your low point of the day. Select a pure, relatively unprocessed carbohydrate, like crackers or fruit, that doesn't have any added appeal in terms of fat or refined sugar. See if your mood and energy seem to improve in the hour or two after eating. Even if you consider yourself a carbohydrate craver, take a close look at what you're eating to see if it actually has the potential to increase brain serotonin production. Is your usual breakfast cereal with milk? An Egg McMuffin? There is probably too much protein in these breakfasts to give you a serotonin-based boost.

In place of your usual mixed-carbo food choices, experiment with choosing a pure carbohydrate meal or snack at the times of day when your energy or mood tends to sag, or when you are most tempted by a high-fat or high-sugar binge food. For most people with serotonin-related symptoms, dinner is the best meal for meeting your daily protein requirements.

Healthy Serotonin-Enhancing Alternatives:

Breakfast:
- Toast, bagel, brioche, or English muffin with fruit preserves or a tiny dab of cream cheese or butter
- Dry cereal and orange juice
- Whole-grain muffin and juice or fruit
- Fruit salad

Lunch:
- Salads
- Vegetarian stir-fry or noodle dishes such as ramen
- Meatless, low cheese pasta dishes
- Veggie sandwiches

Snacks:
- Fresh fruit salad or banana
- Raisins or other dried fruit (small quantities)
- Plain or lightly salted popcorn
- Graham crackers with no added sugar
- Bread, crackers, or whole-grain muffins
- Baked, not fried, chips
- Lightly salted pretzels

Not your personal favorites? All the better! A study done by Dr. John Blundell found that people became hungry again faster after consuming a meal consisting of highly preferred foods than after eating less preferred foods containing an equal number of calories. In other words, the foods we crave are the ones most likely to be followed by renewed hunger.

Even if these alternatives are less overwhelmingly appealing to you than your usual treats, tell yourself you will try anything "just once." See if you have better mood and symptom control in the next couple of hours after your pure carbohydrate food. You may be a true carbohydrate lover who was looking for nourishment in all the wrong food groups!

9

Foods to Feel Good: The High-Carbohydrate Approach to Boosting Serotonin

We must eat to live, and we are compelled to eat by hunger. Yet in our society of abundance, we most often eat for pleasure, in order to feel good. When we are truly hungry, any food will do. When, on the other hand, we seek food to satisfy our feelings, only a few select foods may please us. We tend to suppose our food cravings and preferences reflect our biological needs. In fact, most of us are poorly equipped by instinct alone to pick the foods that satisfy our physiological needs *and* improve our mood and energy state. We might choose well for ourselves if we lived in a traditional society and raised most of our own food. Instead, we are constantly tempted by manufactured high-fat, high-sugar foods that have been given every possible "choose-me" allurement of taste, smell, texture, and appearance—even including psychologist-tested, focus-group-approved packaging. To suppose that we would naturally choose the most wholesome feel-good foods is like imagining that a young man who came into a room full of supermodels and actresses seeking a loving, supportive companion would realize that the quiet brunette with the glasses was the right woman for him. In fact, our food cravings may sometimes serve to make symptoms worse. Some migraine sufferers, for example, crave the very foods that will bring on another migraine attack.

The chemistry of food and mood is not well understood, beyond the established role of serotonin and possible contributions of the endorphins. There may be significant differences between individuals, since some seem to find carbohydrates energizing while others are sedated by them. This chapter serves to give you general information on food-mood connections, so you can scrutinize your own cravings and tastes to see if they are, in fact, hurting or helping any serotonin-related symptoms you may have.

Although we will discuss only the effects of food on mood in this chapter, it is reasonable to assume that other serotonin-related symptoms are affected in similar ways. In fact, the high-carbohydrate, serotonin-friendly diet avoids many known migraine triggers and generally conforms to the dietary recommendations given to headache sufferers. Binge eaters and overeaters will find that paying attention to the impact of food on their mood-energy state will help them manage their eating by choosing foods that will give them better appetite satisfaction and control.

We will not claim that every food-mood connection is mediated directly by serotonin. The list of neurotransmitters and hormones known to influence mood, energy, appetite, pleasure, and pain is long and still growing. On a practical level, if you are able to choose your foods and activities so that you feel better and more energetic, with improved control over your appetite, impulses, and pain conditions, it hardly matters whether the scientific explanation is "serotonin" or "serotonin, endorphins, norepinephrine, dopamine, and factors x, y, and z that we don't know much about yet." If you make lifestyle changes that give you a more stable, positive mood and energy state, plus enhanced self-control and pain tolerance, the cumulative benefit can be assumed to include stabilizing and enhancing the activity of your brain's serotonin system.

Use what this chapter tells you about food and mood to explore your own responses and to experiment with how changes in what you eat and when you eat can improve how you feel and perform.

Sugar, Insulin, and Mood

Sugar can give an energy boost comparable to caffeine. Sugar brings a burst of fast-burning energy that may be responsible for the craving so many people have for high-sugar snacks and breakfasts. For many people, though, a sugar high is followed by a sugar low, even a sugar crash, two or three hours later. Some people will get jittery or nauseous after consuming larger than usual amounts of sugar. It has been implicated in hyperactivity in children, though the connection is controversial. Sugar does seem to have quasi-addictive qualities, since anyone accustomed to a sweet snack or beverage at a certain hour of the day finds it very difficult to do without, or to pass up dessert even after a large meal. We clearly seek sugar not just for taste but for mood-enhancing qualities and its quick-energy effects.

A meal or snack that is high in sugar may raise energy and mood, but there may be a payback later for this quick and easy boost. Whenever any form of sugar is digested and enters the bloodstream, it triggers the release of insulin.

Processed sugar or sucrose is rapidly broken down (metabolized) into glucose, the form in which the body uses sugar. A highly sugary snack will result in the release of large amounts of glucose within a very short time, triggering a surge in insulin release by the pancreas. Although starch is categorized as a complex carbohydrate, foods high in refined flours also produce a sudden insulin burst—sometimes more than candy!

Insulin serves to regulate the amount of glucose in the bloodstream and its uptake by the body's tissues. When blood sugar rises, increased insulin release will cause the tissues to take up the glucose and the liver to store it in the form of glycogen. As the sugar is rapidly removed from the bloodstream, there can be a rebound effect two to four hours later, which will make you hungry again, even though you have had more than enough calories to get by. Apparently, the pancreas "predicts" another large dose of sugar and releases a surge of insulin in expectation—driving the blood sugar level quite low. You will quickly become irritable, hungry, and weak. This response is sometimes called reactive hypoglycemia to indicate that it is different from true hypoglycemia, in which there is a metabolic disorder causing the drop in blood sugar. During the sugar low that follows the sugar high, susceptible individuals may get symptoms of hypoglycemia if they resist the renewed hunger pangs. These include dizziness, shakiness, anxiety, nausea, sweating, and rapid heartbeat—all the fight-or-flight symptoms that here serve to alert you to eat, and soon! Eating again will rapidly restore normal blood sugar and the symptoms will disappear.

Migraine sufferers often have headaches triggered by a sudden drop in blood sugar. For this reason, they are generally advised to avoid foods high in refined sugar, corn syrup, or honey. Although honey is popularly considered to be a healthy and natural sweetener, commercial honeybees are fed large amounts of sugar and corn syrup to increase honey production. Honey-sweetened granola bars and cookies are just as likely to send you on a sugar-fueled roller coaster ride as a Snickers bar or a bag of jelly beans.

If you like sweet snacks as your serotonin boost, try fresh fruit instead, which is more slowly converted by the body to glucose. When you drink a glass of orange juice or munch on an apple, a small amount of the fruit sugar, called fructose, is absorbed directly into the bloodstream from the digestive tract, giving you a modest but noticeable energy boost. However, the rest of the fructose is converted to glucose in the liver relatively slowly, so the insulin release is relatively low. Depending on the type of fruit, this may not be sufficient to provide a serotonin-mediated mood lift, but some people will benefit by using a fruit as a sweet treat that provides energy without destabilizing blood sugar. Combining a starch with a fruit snack might provide the best energy and mood-food combination.

The sucrose sugars, including refined sugars, corn syrup, honey, and other sweeteners, consist of a double sugar molecule made up of glucose plus fructose. In the digestive tract, the glucose is rapidly separated from fructose and released into the bloodstream, triggering a big insulin surge within just a few minutes. With a fruit snack you avoid the rapid swings in blood sugar that bring you momentarily high only to send your crashing a few hours later. Canned fruit to which sugar has been added and dried fruit such as raisins in which sugar is more concentrated may also trigger reactive hypoglycemia in some people. People who are prone to episodes of reactive hypoglycemia may benefit by eating a number of small "nibble" meals throughout the day, plus a carbohydrate snack at bedtime. There are often mood and binge-avoidance benefits from doing so as well.

Mood, Minerals, and Vitamins

Poor dietary habits are common in depressed persons. They may be occurring as a result of the depression, yet they may well be helping to perpetuate it. The same may be said for the nutritional deficiencies that frequently accompany eating disorders, migraine, insomnia, and PMS. Deficiencies in B complex vitamins, vitamin C, niacin, and folic acid have been found to accompany mental illness. Even borderline deficiencies of vitamins B_1, B_2, B_6, and niacin are associated with irritability, nervousness, fatigue, mental confusion, depression, and emotional instability.

The significance of vitamins for mood and mental functioning has not been extensively studied, despite the fact that a number of vitamins are known to be necessary for the production of important neurotransmitters and hormones. For example, pyridoxal phosphate, a derivative of vitamin B_6, is needed to produce norepinephrine and serotonin. An inadequate intake of vitamin B_6, necessary for the formation of serotonin, has been associated with insomnia, irritability, and depression. Vitamin B complex is used in a supplemental treatment for insomnia, migraine, and PMS. Interestingly, women on oral contraceptives often have lower blood levels of thiamin, riboflavin, B_6, B_{12}, and vitamin C, and depression can occur as a side effect of the pill, presumably as a result of B_6 deficiency plus estrogen-influenced fluctuation in serotonin. Heavy alcohol drinkers are also deficient in thiamin and vitamin B_6. Iron and vitamin C also play a part in serotonin synthesis, as well as in so many other essential physiological processes. Niacin deficiencies are considered by some physicians to have a role in depression and alcoholism, but this has not yet been confirmed by careful study.

You can certainly consider taking vitamin supplements, though choosing natural sources is always preferable. Megadoses of vitamin B_6 have been reported to create dependency, so that depression and other symptoms of B_6 deficiency can result if supplementation is reduced or stopped. For this reason, unless you are following your doctor's advice, you should not take more than 50–100 mg daily, the amount contained in many supplements, which is far in excess of the recommended daily allowance (RDA) of 2 mg. In fact, you should be getting adequate amounts of vitamin B_6 by following the serotonin-friendly dietary guidelines. Whole grains and fresh or frozen vegetables and fruits are the best sources. Because B_6 is a water-soluble vitamin, some proportion of it is lost in cooking. Drained canned fruits and vegetables may have lost as much as 90 percent of their vitamin B_6 content.

Mood and Cholesterol? An Unexplained Mystery

As everyone knows, high blood cholesterol levels are a major risk factor for heart attack and other cardiovascular disease. We have all been urged to limit consumption of animal fat and trans fats. Millions of people are now taking cholesterol-lowering drugs such as Mevacor (lovastatin), Zocor (simvastatin), and Lescol (fluvastatin) to reduce the amount of cholesterol in the bloodstream, in order to prevent deposits of cholesterol from forming in blood vessels. Sounds like good sense and good medicine, yet a 1990 British study that pooled the results of several studies on the long-term survival of men taking cholesterol-lowering drugs produced some surprising results. These men did in fact have reduced mortality from heart disease compared to another group of men who did not take an anticholesterol medication. However, that benefit was wiped out by the fact that the men taking the medication had a higher rate of death due to accidents, suicide, or violence. The difference was substantial, and the number of men involved was so large (nearly 25,000) that this unexpected finding couldn't be dismissed as a statistical blip. It occasioned much debate and additional studies designed to confirm or disprove a link between low cholesterol and increased aggression or impulsiveness.

It was possible that the higher incidence of accidents and violence might be an unknown side effect of the drugs themselves, not related to the reduction in cholesterol levels. For this reason, researchers have begun to look at the effects of low-cholesterol diets on animals. One such study, led by Dr. Jay Kaplan, compared the behavior of two groups of monkeys, one on a high-cholesterol diet and the other group on a low-cholesterol (yet high-fat) diet. The researchers found that monkeys on the lower cholesterol diet had signs of reduced serotonin activity (lower levels of metabolites in their spinal fluid). Their behavior, assessed by independent observers, was more aggressive and antisocial than that of the other group of monkeys. Another study by Dr. Kaplan's group compared the effects of high-fat, high-cholesterol and low-fat, low-cholesterol diets. In this case also the monkeys on a low-cholesterol diet were more aggressive and had indicators of lower serotonin system activity.

Yet another study examined cholesterol level in 650 patients hospitalized for psychiatric illnesses and compared it to their history of suicide attempts. There was a correlation. Men with low cholesterol levels (25th percentile or less) were twice as likely to have made a serious suicide attempt at some point in their lives. Other studies surveying the general population have also found higher rates of suicide among men (not women) with low cholesterol levels. In studies of boys and men with histories of criminal conduct, there were associations between aggression and lower cholesterol levels.

These studies do *not* indicate that you should slather huge amounts of butter on bread and baked potatoes, or eat fried foods with abandon.

No one yet knows for certain how cholesterol levels might affect serotonin synthesis or activity. One of cholesterol's known functions is to help produce the insulating sheath that surrounds nerve fibers, allowing them to transmit their messages. Until there is a testable theory or mechanism to explain how cholesterol might affect mood, or much more evidence indicating that the link is real, the risk of heart disease from too much cholesterol must be considered more significant than the risk of accidents or out-of-control aggression. Your best good mood and good health strategy would be to eat animal fat and shortening, which raise blood cholesterol, in moderation, particularly if you are subject to irritable bowel syndrome. However, foods that act to reduce the levels of LDL (low-density lipoprotein) or bad cholesterol in the bloodstream may offer both mood and health benefits. These include vegetable oils, such as olive oil, and the oils contained in nuts and seeds such as sesame, safflower, sunflower, and peanut.

Mood and Dietary Fat

We crave fat in the form of fried and buttery foods just as we crave sugar, but do the high-fat foods we love return our affection by improving mood and energy? The answer may vary from individual to individual. Studies of the impact of fat consumption on serotonin and mood have indicated no effects or slightly negative effects, despite the fact that on a long-term basis, cholesterol may be needed for serotonin functioning. It is perhaps important to know that most of the body's cholesterol is synthesized by the liver, so dietary cholesterol does not necessarily determine whether a given individual's cholesterol level is high or low. Someone might have low cholesterol, low serotonin, and a tendency to impulsiveness or violence while consuming eggs, bacon, and thickly buttered toast every day!

Fat slows the digestion, and most people will find that a high-fat meal will leave them feeling sluggish—relaxed and calmed perhaps, but much less physically active and mentally alert. Because of the slowed-down digestion of food, a carbohydrate that includes a considerable amount of fat will have a slower and more modest effect on increasing the supply of tryptophan to the brain. Studies by Dr. John Blundell, among others, have suggested that high-fat meals do not have the appetite-satisfying effects often claimed for them, whereas high-carbohydrate meals do. This, too, may vary greatly from individual to individual. In keeping your Mood-Food-Activity Journal, consider also how the fat content of meals—high, moderate, or low—might be affecting your mood and symptoms.

Mood and Caffeine

Along with alcohol, caffeine ranks as one of the most popular mood modulators in general use. As a stimulant, caffeine has quite significant effects on wakefulness and attention. Many people reach for caffeine when their mood is down for the sake of this pick-me-up effect, yet a sudden increase in caffeine intake can have a very unpleasant effect. Excessive caffeine will induce anxiety-like symptoms (coffee nerves), such as trembling, a hyperalert state, and a quickened heart rate. In susceptible individuals these symptoms can contribute to a state of chronic anxiety or even a full-blown panic attack. Often we are so accustomed to using it to bring our energy (or sobriety) back up that caffeine's effects on mood are not noticed or are tolerated for the sake of its wake-up call.

For people prone to insomnia, late afternoon caffeine intake can disturb sleep. A high daily intake of caffeine is also implicated in chronic headache problems, despite the fact that well-timed doses of caffeine can be used as a headache treatment. Unfortunately, caffeine withdrawal also causes headaches. Whether caffeine has any positive or negative effects on serotonin system activity has not been demonstrated, though some claims and guesses have been put forward. Recovering alcoholics often become heavy coffee drinkers, suggesting that caffeine is sought for mood-modulating effects, but this does not necessarily mean it affects serotonin release. More likely, coffee jitters can be a welcome distraction from a depressed, low-energy mood, and the person recovering from alcohol abuse still has the impulse to keep drinking something.

Mood and Food Additives

Monosodium glutamate (MSG) has been known to have potentially toxic effects for decades, ever since the first reports of "Chinese restaurant syndrome," in which large amounts of MSG added to food were found to trigger headaches, trembling, and sweating. Today, however, MSG is less heavily used in Chinese restaurants, due to all the bad press. Yet it is now found in almost all processed, nonfresh foods, whether canned or frozen, containing meat, fish, or vegetables. The average American consumes about one-third of a pound of MSG per year. A little here and a little there may not have any ill effects on the average person. However, MSG is a known migraine trigger, and even small doses will bring on a migraine attack in susceptible individuals.

The effects of MSG are thought to result from the fact that glutamate is another one of the brain's neurotransmitters. The consumption of large doses of MSG could potentially raise the levels of glutamate in the brain and modify its functioning. Experiments with animals given huge doses of MSG have not confirmed the theory. If you are prone to headaches, you should watch for signs that your headaches might be triggered by MSG-containing foods.

The artificial sweetener aspartame (Equal, Nutrasweet) has also been suspected of affecting brain function by increasing the availability of aspartate, another neurotransmitter. Animal studies have not confirmed a link between the aspartate contained in the sweetener and any measurable changes in the brain. Yet it is also a reported migraine trigger, though a less common one than MSG. Headache sufferers should watch their consumption of aspartame to see if there is an association with their headache attacks. If you tend to binge on sweets and are trying to switch to healthier carbohydrate choices, it is generally a good idea to avoid artificial sweeteners as well. If you rely on artificial sweeteners to satisfy your craving for sugar, you will just be perpetuating your binge problem and risking a relapse. In fact, Leeds researcher John Blundell compared the effects of a midday snack of plain yogurt or artificially sweetened yogurt on calorie intake at a lunch served one hour later. Study participants who were served the plain yogurt consumed a smaller lunch, suggesting that artificial sweeteners do not depress appetite, as often claimed, but in fact stimulate it.

Instead of artificially sweetened beverages, try drinking spring water, flavored seltzer, sparkling water, or unfiltered fruit juice (not sugar-added fruit drinks). If you cut back on both sugar and artificial sweeteners, you may well find, after a month or two, that your old favorite indulgences are now much too sweet for your well-adjusted taste buds.

Mood and Meal Size

The amount of food consumed at a time also has a pronounced effect on mood and energy. Large meals are sedating—a benefit, perhaps, for people who are anxious and a likely motive for bingeing. If you want to emphasize daytime alertness and energy, try consuming several small carbohydrate meals during the day and a reasonable-sized protein and carbohydrate dinner in the evening. There are a number of potential health benefits to multiple small meals versus the traditional two or three square meals. For example, you are likely to achieve better appetite control and more stable blood sugar levels. Experimenting with multiple small meals may help you get a better look at how specific foods affect your mood and other serotonin-related symptoms.

Mood and Protein

There is considerable variation in response to protein versus carbohydrate consumption in terms of mood and alertness. In general, people who identify themselves as carbohydrate cravers and who have serotonin deficiency symptoms will report that protein makes them sleepy while carbohydrates provide energy and mood lifts. Other people will have quite the opposite response. For them, carbohydrates are relaxing and sedating, while protein improves energy and alertness.

If you have symptoms suggesting a serotonin system deficiency, it is likely that you will find carbohydrates energizing and protein sedating. In fact, in studies with both humans and animals, diets or drugs that reduce brain tryptophan levels will tend to increase carbohydrate consumption—suggesting that we do "self-medicate" serotonin deficiencies with carbohydrate foods. On the other hand, diets and drugs that act to increase brain serotonin levels will tend to result in decreased carbohydrate consumption and increased protein and fat consumption. These effects are not universally true, but have been observed in many studies with animals and humans and have been taken as support for the theory that serotonin-deficient individuals self-medicate by increasing carbohydrate consumption. Perhaps people who respond more positively to protein consumption have adequate brain serotonin levels, and increased serotonin is sedating.

People who have already elevated insulin levels may be carbohydrate sensitive and at risk for excessive levels of serum cholesterol and triglyceride (fat) in response to a highly refined diet that includes too much high fructose corn syrup. Don't use the carbohydrate craving theory as a justification for highly processed snacks and sweets. Remember that some recent research described in chapter 8 suggests that "protein avoiding" may be more effective than "carbohydrate seeking" as a mood-elevating strategy for your daytime meals and snacks. If this is the case, then vegan cuisine—just fruits, vegetables, and whole grains—may be the best choice for your low mood times.

To find out how your moods are affected by your foods, you should experiment with the effects of high-protein–low-carbohydrate meals versus high-carbohydrate–low-protein foods, using a Food-Mood-Activity Journal, as described in chapter 12, to record and analyze the mood and energy effects of different foods. You will then know how to distribute your protein and carbohydrate consumption over the course of the day—perhaps having your energizing foods earlier in the day and sedating foods for your evening meal. Each person is bound to have individual quirks in terms of chemistry and metabolism—what's pickles to me is ice cream to you! Even if you do not fit the carbo craving model of the person who experiences a definite lift from carbohydrate consumption, you can use the information in chapters 8, 9, and 12 to help you understand the impact of food on mood, so you have more control over how you feel, behave, and perform.

Picking the Right Carbohydrates

The term "carbohydrate" is commonly used to designate foods ranging in nutritional quality from jelly beans to green beans, cookies to cauliflower, pastries to pears. Carbohydrates are energy foods that provide sugars or starches that the body can burn for instant energy or store in the form of glycogen. The junk varieties of carbohydrates provide little nutrition beyond fuel (so-called empty calories), plus some undesirable saturated fats—the "bad cholesterol" kind. The natural sources can fulfill just about every nutrient you need—providing essential vitamins, minerals, and trace elements, plus fiber to speed digestion and avoid bowel disease. Properly combined and balanced, carbohydrates can also provide all the protein you need, which is vastly less than most Americans consume.

Carbohydrates come in two forms. Simple carbohydrates are those that contain some combination of the sugars glucose, fructose, and sucrose. Complex carbohydrates contain sugars combined into a larger starch molecule. In general, fruits and vegetables are classified as simple carbohydrates, though they may also contain starches, and grains (including pastas, bread, and rice) are considered complex carbohydrates. Simple carbohydrates provide energy lifts as well as essential nutrients. Complex carbohydrates give a longer burning fuel supply, with stick-to-your-ribs power to ward off a return of between-meal appetite. Because these foods also contain a great deal of fiber, they take longer to eat and are more satisfying to eat, while yielding fewer calories than food made from refined sugar and flour. High-fiber carbohydrate diets offer so many health benefits that they are recommended for everyone from athletes to heart disease and diabetes patients. The same foods are also believed, on the basis of considerable evidence, to protect against many types of cancer.

Carbohydrate craving for people with SAD or bingeing problems is often associated with weight gain. However, in these cases the carbohydrates preferred often tend to be highly processed junk carbohydrates, or large portions of starch combined with excess meat and fat. By sticking to low-fat, low-sugar carbohydrates, particularly those that are unprocessed and close to their natural state, you will feel better and be more likely to maintain a steady weight or have a gradual long-term weight loss.

A combination of fruit and cereal for breakfast and a lunch of vegetables and starch (bread, rice, pasta, potatoes, or grains), with fruit for between-meal snacks is a serotonin-friendly diet that will keep your mood up and your appetite down and yield truly impressive health benefits when sustained over time.

The Humble Potato

Despite the low reputation of meat-and-potatoes diets, potatoes themselves are an excellent carbohydrate. It's frying them or adding butter that turns them into high-calorie, high-fat junk. Baked or boiled in their skins, potatoes pack a great deal of nutritional value. Try eating the skin if you do not already do so. It is an excellent source of nutrients.

Whole-Wheat Breads, Crackers, and Muffins

Refined (white) flour has lost much of its B vitamins. Enriched flour adds back some of the lost vitamins, but not vitamin B_6. Read labels to know what you are buying. Wheat flour is not the same as whole wheat flour. Some crackers contain substantial amounts of added fat and sugar, so check the label for both the total calories and the calories from fat.

Breakfast Cereals

Choose unsweetened, high-fiber oat or whole-grain cereals. The old standards, such as Shredded Wheat, Cheerios, Wheaties, Total, Raisin Bran, All-Bran, and Wheat Chex are all good choices, but avoid the sugared and flavored versions. If you see more than one type of sugar listed among the ingredients, for example, corn syrup, maltose, honey, and dextrose, or if the sugar comes high in the list of ingredients, the total amount of sweetener may be excessive. Whole grains do contain some protein. If the breakfast cereal label indicates that there is more than ten times as much carbohydrate as protein, there is probably too much added sugar from a nutritional standpoint. Whole-grain hot cereals such as cream of wheat, farina, and oatmeal are excellent foods; cook them with water rather than milk to enjoy their serotonin-boosting benefits. Use only a little milk, or try pouring orange juice on your cereal. Most fruit-and-nut granola blends also include a fair amount of protein, particularly if you add milk, so granola may not have the serotonin-increasing effects you need in the morning.

Brown Rice Is Best

Three billion people can't be wrong! Rice is *the* staple for much of the world. It provides modest amounts of protein in addition to essential B vitamins, and as a carbohydrate it is easy to digest. Brown rice retains the vitamin-rich bran and germ, which are removed in the polishing process used to produce white rice. Although white rice is still considered a healthy and nutritious carbohydrate, it has less than half the B_6 of brown rice, and greatly reduced amounts of other B vitamins. Brown rice requires more cooking time but rewards the cook with a rich, nutty flavor. In the current rice renaissance, the adventuresome cook can find dozens of exotic rice varieties in gourmet and natural food stores—some with beautiful colors and delicate flavors that give them stand-alone qualities as side dishes, quite unlike the blandness associated with most supermarket white rice varieties.

Other Great Grains

Bulgur wheat, kasha, quinoa, and couscous are amazingly easy and quick to prepare. To prepare bulgur wheat and couscous, you simply add boiling water and let them sit, covered, for a few minutes. Then season with spices and add nuts, vegetables, diced meat, or poultry. There are literally hundreds of great grain recipes, and reading just a few of them will give you great ideas for adding your own favorite tastes or recycling yesterday's leftovers. Although you can purchase these delicious staples in small, overpriced packages in most supermarkets, if you go to a natural food store that sells them by the pound you can feed your family for pennies. You might try the supermarket versions first, and save the cartons for the recipes and cooking instructions.

Four-Star Staples

Beans, peas, and barley, combined with vegetables and spices, can be the basis of a great variety of wholesome and economical soups and casseroles. Canned beans are time-savers, but quick-cook methods using dried beans can also provide an easy meal made from scratch. Beans in particular are an excellent source of protein when combined with rice or corn. High in iron, low in fat, *and* low in cost, beans are one of the best all-round foods in terms of the number of nutritional needs they satisfy. If you are bothered by flatulence after eating beans, try soaking them longer in larger quantities of water, and add a little baking soda to the soaking water. This problem diminishes for most people who consume beans regularly. As for barley, the more common pearled barley has had the husk and germ removed and is less nutritious than whole hulled barley, found in some health food stores. Both barley and beans have serum cholesterol–lowering effects when consumed regularly.

Popcorn

Unbuttered popcorn is a first-rate nibble food, a favorite of both athletes and weight watchers. There are only twenty-nine calories in a cup of plain popcorn. If you need some seasoning, sprinkle a little salt, a tiny bit of Parmesan, or (if you are not MSG-sensitive) some seasoned salt.

Pasta! Pasta!

With a tomato-based or vegetable sauce rather than a cream sauce, pasta is a good-for-you carbohydrate that appeals to just about everyone. It is widely identified as a comfort food by sufferers from SAD and by binge eaters, suggesting that it might well be sought out for mood-improving qualities. However, pasta itself is about 13 percent protein. If you choose pasta for a serotonin-enhancing meal, you should stick to pasta dishes that contain tomatoes and other vegetables only, with little or no added protein, such as cheese. Most pasta salads and hot pasta dishes with marinara, tomato, or roasted red pepper sauces would be just fine. For your dinner, pasta with a meat sauce, a fish-, cheese- or meat-stuffed ravioli, or just a grating of cheese on top will give you a nicely balanced protein and carbohydrate meal. When you buy pasta for cooking at home, try to get pasta made with 100 percent semolina or durum flour. Or choose whole wheat, spinach, or other vegetable-flavored pastas for variety.

Salads and Raw Veggies

A salad you make or assemble at a salad bar is an excellent simple carbohydrate that is all good news in terms of nutrition and calories, so long as you don't overdress. An oil-and-vinegar dressing is much preferred to a heavy, creamy one, and the really heavy ones, such as blue cheese, should be avoided altogether. If it makes it easier for you, you could put on an oil-and-vinegar–type dressing first, then add a little of a heavier, fattier dressing as a garnish. Buttermilk- and yogurt-based dressings are also good choices, provided you use a light touch when you pour them on.

Fruit Plus Breads: The Mood-Energy Combo

Fruit gives a healthier, more sustained energy boost than a refined-sugar snack such as cookies, pastries, or candy. Fructose or fruit sugar is passively absorbed, so that the increase in insulin release is less extreme. Because of the lower insulin release, the mood benefit of fruit *alone* results largely from stabilizing blood sugar. You are very unlikely to experience reactive hypoglycemia or to have a sudden return in hunger as your blood sugar drops—a frequent consequence of snacks containing much higher quantities of sucrose (refined sugar), honey, or high fructose sweetener. There is a great deal of variation in the fructose and sucrose content of fruit, however. For example, oranges, melons, and peaches contain a relatively high proportion of sucrose, although they are still low-calorie snacks. By releasing more insulin, they may have a greater impact on serotonin supply. Having a whole-grain muffin, graham crackers, or other complex carbo with fruit or unfiltered fruit juice is an excellent combination for providing a rapid but sustained mood and energy lift.

Fruit sugar reaches the bloodstream more quickly than the sugars released from complex carbohydrate, so if your blood sugar is low, you may experience a more rapid improvement in mood and energy—just the thing for midmorning and midafternoon snacks. If you are making the transition from sugary snacks, grapes and bananas make excellent good-for-you substitutes. Apples, oranges, and grapefruits are good almost all year round; grapes and pears are great in the fall; berries, peaches, and melons are best eaten during the summer.

Carbohydrates and Glycemic Index

The glycemic index compares the amount of glucose released into the blood by specific foods. It offers a ballpark estimate as to how greatly a specific carbohydrate will trigger an insulin surge, thereby increasing the supply of tryptophan to the brain. The higher the glycemic index, the greater the insulin release is likely to be.

As you use the chart on page 201 for reference in designing serotonin-friendly meal and snack choices, remember that a varied, well-balanced diet is the best mood and energy enhancer of all. *Do not over-select from high glycemic index foods.* Excessive consumption of foods high on the glycemic index is linked to the development of metabolic syndrome and insulin resistance—both of them risk factors for adult-onset diabetes. Obesity is the number one risk factor for adult-onset diabetes, so this association may reflect only the inevitable weight gain of people who indulge too heavily in sugary or starchy foods. In either case, donuts and candy bars may be very effective in achieving a brief mood boost, but they are hardly good staples for long-term health and happiness. The insulin surge triggered by high glycemic index foods is often followed by an abrupt drop in insulin two to three hours later, which will leave you with a famished craving for another snack and perhaps a mood drop as well.

Understand, however, that the glycemic index is simply a guide, and a very rough one at that. Rarely does anyone sit down to a meal consisting of white rice and nothing but white rice. (Unless they are subjects in a laboratory experiment!) The glycemic index of mixed foods or meals is not well researched. Different varieties of a food, prepared different ways, can have different GI values. Boiled red potatoes served hot have a higher glycemic index value (89) than the same potatoes served cold (56) because cooked starches gelatinize (harden) into a less digestible form when they cool. The same would be true for hot pasta versus cold pasta in a salad, or bread fresh out of the oven compared to completely cooled

THE GLYCEMIC INDEX FOR COMMON FOODS
(BASED ON GLUCOSE=100)

Glycemic Index	Cereals/Grains/ Starches	Vegetables	Fruit

70–87%	instant rice
	baked potato
	rice cakes
	white bread
	corn flakes
	unsweetened
	  breakfast
	  cereals
		none	watermelon

50%–70%	whole wheat
	  bread
	sourdough
	  bread
	pumpernickel
	white rice
	brown rice
	new potatoes
	corn meal
	oatmeal
		corn
		sweet potato
		parsnips
		beets
		carrots
			bananas
			raisins
			papayas
			mangoes

30%–50%	pasta converted rice bran cereal	peas pinto beans garbanzo beans	oranges apples pears
20%–30%	barley	lentils kidney beans lima beans soy beans	peaches grapefruit

bread. Also, the specific types of sugar or starch have different effects on blood sugar. Even plain old white bread varies considerably, depending on the proportions of high glycemic (amylopectin) and low glycemic (amylose) starches in the flour used to make it. More spectacularly, different varieties of rice (containing different proportions of starch and cooked by different methods—values for parboiled or converted rice are lower because of starch gelatinization) can range from 33 to 109 on the glycemic index. Finally, although it is a very popular concept in some currently fashionable diet plans, the glycemic index does not distinguish "healthy" from "unhealthy" foods. Table sugar has a modest GI of 65. Tofu frozen desserts have an extremely high glycemic index (115) compared to good old ice cream (35 for French vanilla). Rather than eat by the numbers, pay attention to how your energy level and your mood are affected for the two or three hours after a meal or snack. That will tell you far more than calorie counts, glycemic index comparisons, or food composition percentages!

If you find by your own experience that high glycemic index foods are more effective in raising your moods, then tiny servings at your low mood moments may be a good option; they will produce a quick but small surge in blood sugar that is less likely to result in excessive fluctuations in insulin levels. Go ahead and have those jelly beans (GI=80), but just a few at a time. If you are committed to a healthy diet and not all that tempted by sweet treats, try a glass of orange juice. It has just enough sucrose to produce a rapid but modest rise in blood sugar.

Once again, if you have a tendency to fill up (or binge) on highly refined carbohydrates, do not misread or misuse the information in this book as justifying your diet as healthy or as necessary for your mood. The relationship between insulin, blood sugar level, and mood is quite complex and not yet well understood. On a short-term basis, a high glycemic index food that raises the insulin level will also raise serotonin availability in the brain. On a chronic basis, consuming highly refined carbohydrates as a major source of calories may have negative effects on both physical and mental well-being. Depression is twice as common in people with diabetes compared to nondiabetics, and those with poorly controlled blood sugar levels have the highest incidence of depression. There is also some evidence to support the reverse correlation: People with major depression are more likely to be insulin resistant and so at risk of developing diabetes.

Will I Get Enough Protein?

The average American consumes twice as much protein as needed, and that extra protein usually gets converted to fat. Since vegetables and complex carbohydrates do contain some protein, two ounces of animal protein per serving in your evening meal in the form of dairy, fish, poultry, or meat will amply meet the protein needs of an average adult. If you feel that less than a half pound is skimping, experiment with increasing the grain, bean, and vegetable content of your meals and cutting the animal protein. Try cutting back an ounce at a time. You may be surprised by how much more alert you feel in the evening. Reducing excess protein consumption can help make your weekday evenings quality time rather than conk-out time. If your family judges the appeal of a meal by the size of the slab of meat put on their plate, try out some one-dish casseroles that combine vegetables, complex carbohydrates, and moderate portions of animal protein.

Strict vegan vegetarians do need to pay attention to protein requirements (as well as vitamin B_{12}) when they plan their meals because the protein found in most plant foods is incomplete, lacking one or more essential amino acids. They have to be sure they combine plant foods that together provide all the needed amino acids, not necessarily at every meal, but over the course of a day. Nuts and beans are good protein sources, especially when combined with a grain. Many traditional meals that serve legumes (beans) with grains such as rice or corn meet this requirement perfectly; so does spreading peanut butter on crackers or bread. If you add dairy products such as cheese or include eggs, fish, or small amounts of poultry and meat in your diet, you do not need to worry about getting enough protein. You will likely benefit by not getting too much!

Where to Begin—Some Sample Menus

Menu No. 1. Start the Day Strong

Mood Boosting Breakfast
> Cereal, dry or with ½ cup milk; fruit or juice
> *or*
> Brioche, toast or muffin, preserves, fruit or juice

Keep Up the Good Mood Lunch
> Pasta primavera or pasta salad
> *or*
> Tossed spring mixed salad, mixed vegetable salad, or classic Caesar salad (no chicken or other added protein)

Late Day Energy Snack
> Apple and graham crackers

Relax with Dinner
> 4-ounce serving of meat, fish, or dairy protein source with balanced selection of vegetables and starch

Menu No. 2. Beat Winter Blahs

Warm-up Breakfast
> Cream of wheat or oatmeal
> *or*
> French toast and fruit

Snack If You Need It
Banana or raisins

High-Comfort Lunch
French bread pizza
or
Vegetable-bean soup with bread

Afternoon Mood Lift
Irish soda bread (if available), pretzels (remove excess salt), or cinnamon-raisin bagel with preserves

Light and Mellow Dinner
Stir-fry with rice
or
Pasta with hearty tomato sauce

Menu No. 3. Light, Cool, and Buoyant

No Time to Eat Breakfast
Glass of orange juice—a healthy way to get a quick sugar boost

Or, Natural Energy Breakfast
Fruit salad with ⅓ cup plain or flavored yogurt

Mostly Green Lunch
Cool summer soup (gazpacho, cucumber, etc.) with whole wheat or rye bread
or
Veggie sandwich on whole wheat pita

Light and Satisfying Dinner
Quiche and salad or raw vegetables
or

Chef's salad

or

Salad niçoise (tuna, green beans, olives, potatoes)

As you try these sample menus (or your own favorite carbo combos), keep a Food-Mood-Activity Journal, as described in chapter 12, to track your success in minimizing serotonin-related symptoms. By carefully timing your carbohydrate and protein intake, you can identify the food combinations that will help you feel and function at your best—all day, throughout the month, and year round.

10

Jogging Works, but So Does Chewing Gum!

Exercise is a well-known antidepressant. Study after study has shown that the incidence of depression is lower among people who exercise regularly, compared to nonexercisers matched for age, income, and other socioeconomic factors. While it is true that extremely depressed people are often too overwhelmed to get out of bed, much less jog around the park, both studies and case reports indicate that regular—better yet, daily—exercise is an excellent treatment for depression and anxiety. The mood-elevating effects of exercise last for about four hours, long enough for people with only mild-to-moderate mood problems to shift their focus away from any sad or anxious preoccupations to positive and productive concerns, such as work, socializing, and taking care of house and family.

The mood-enhancing effects of running have been the most studied and discussed. Yet more moderate exercise, including swimming and walking, appears to have comparable benefits. A study conducted at the University of Wisconsin found that a twelve-week exercise program (in this case jogging) with a trainer is as effective in alleviating moderate depression as twelve weeks of either traditional or time-limited psychotherapy. What's more, the moderately depressed people in the exercise program achieved better long-term results. When they were evaluated one year later, the exercisers were still jogging and were free of depression, while 50 percent of those treated by psychotherapy were still in treatment or had returned for more treatment. Apparently, the people treated with psychotherapy received empathy, insight, and understanding that helped them in the short term, but the exercise group had acquired a coping and self-help skill that ultimately served them better.

Exercise: Is It Endorphins or Serotonin?

The feel-good effects of exercise have often been attributed to endorphins, the body's natural opium-like tranquilizers. Yet studies show that brain endorphin release is not dramatically increased except with a level of exertion and exhaustion few of us undertake. It requires running a full marathon to bring on a true runner's high, which is a trancelike state of euphoria. In experiments in which the effects of endorphins were blocked by drug treatment, healthy volunteers reported that they still experienced a relaxed and elevated mood after finishing their workout.

People who exercise regularly in moderation—walking, running, swimming, cycling, aerobics, or working out at a gym—find that their workout reliably elevates their mood without making them either fatigued or euphoric. Rather, they are left relaxed, focused, and alert. Contrary to popular beliefs among couch potatoes, most people who exercise regularly (daily or on alternate days) year in, year out, are not motivated so much by the desire to control their weight or improve their health. These are negatively defined goals, in which a person is avoiding a punishment rather than seeking a reward. Rather, they stick with their exercise program because they get very real pleasure from it—the kind of mood lift that nonexercisers seek (and do not find) from caffeine, alcohol, and high-sugar, high-fat foods. Moderate to vigorous exercise will release tension, counteract depressed or anxious feelings, and combat food and alcohol cravings. It is also a key recommendation of most pain-control programs and experts.

During exercise, endorphins are released by the nerves supplying the muscles. They act to limit the painful effects of muscle exertion. These endorphins don't cross into the brain, however, but stay in the body, so they do not affect mood. Instead, the upbeat mood induced by exercise is more likely to be the result of norepinephrine and serotonin release, with some contribution from brain endorphins. One laboratory study showed a doubling of brain serotonin levels in animals exercised on a treadmill for ninety minutes. Another study indicated that regular exercise produces an increase in brain serotonin production and activity in animals that lasts for weeks after exercise is discontinued.

Exercise has so many mental and physiological benefits that there is no reason to focus on its effects on serotonin system functioning, even though these might be central to its antidepressant qualities. Michael H. Sacks, a dedicated runner and a psychiatrist at Weill-Cornell Medical College, suggests that several factors may contribute to the positive impact of exercise on mood, including:

- Making the decision to take up exercise—many depressed or anxious people feel better after their first exercise effort
- The symbolic meaning of the activity—"I'm doing something to help myself; I'm going to be healthier"
- The distraction from worries
- The pleasure of mastery of a sport
- The positive self-image
- The physiological effects—improved cardiovascular tone, stamina, muscle strength, posture, digestion, and metabolism, etc.
- The biochemical effects—increases in serotonin, norepinephrine, and endorphin activity, and perhaps other brain and nervous system changes we don't yet know about.

Exercise: A Win-Win and Win-Big Situation

Increasing serotonin activity and controlling serotonin-related symptoms are only the latest good news about the benefits of exercise. The more familiar still apply. Exercise is the most effective long-term approach to weight control. Vigorous exercise gives an immediate calorie burn of 200–300 calories for a thirty-minute aerobic workout. Just as important, exercise sets your body's metabolic rate higher for up to fifteen hours after your workout. So you continue to burn more calories for the rest of the day—at the same time feeling more alert, energetic, and productive. People who are very fit and active consume about 600 calories more a day, yet weigh 20 percent less than their inactive peers, partly because muscle tissue is metabolically very active, so it needs more calories both during activity and at rest.

Regular exercise lowers serum cholesterol levels and reduces blood pressure. People who exercise regularly have lower resting pulse rates yet can safely and easily double their pulse rate during an aerobic workout. A strengthened heart pumps more blood with less effort. Exercise strengthens bones and prevents osteoporosis. And exercise helps control and possibly prevent diabetes by increasing the utilization of blood sugar. Finally, exercising outdoors increases your exposure to natural light, a significant mood enhancer for people with SAD or bad weather moods.

Serotonin and Movement

Barry Jacobs is a neuroscience researcher at Princeton University who performs highly exacting studies of serotonin functioning in laboratory animals. He has devoted his career to understanding how serotonin activity in specific areas of the brains of animals is involved in the animal's awareness and activity level. Although analyzing rat brain extracts would appear to be a long way from understanding why human beings feel anxious or sad or overeat, his studies have great relevance to understanding how exercise can promote serotonin functioning.

Dr. Jacobs's research is based on the observation that serotonin is found in the nervous systems of all vertebrates (animals with internal skeletons, from fish to humans) and in many primitive animals, such as the humble garden slug. Therefore, it must have some important fundamental function, in addition to more complex mood and behavior regulation. The most basic function of brain serotonin appears to be motor control—regulating the fundamental yet all-important ability to move at will.

In a number of experiments with laboratory animals, Dr. Jacobs discovered that there is a clear relationship between brain serotonin system activity and movement. In the motor control areas of the brain, serotonin nerve cells are active throughout the waking day. As noted in chapter 2, serotonin activity shuts down dramatically during REM sleep, the dreaming part of the sleep cycle when the sleeper is paralyzed by a temporary loss of tone in key muscles. By administering drugs that induce temporary paralysis in wide-awake animals, his research team discovered that serotonin activity was nearly completely suppressed during the paralysis. These results suggest serotonin activity is closely linked with movement, and with the muscle tone necessary for movement.

In yet another set of studies, Dr. Jacobs's research group found that serotonin activity increases by a factor of two to five when an animal is engaged in repetitive movements involving the mouth. These include biting, chewing, or grooming the fur with the tongue, as well as the expectation of eating. This increase might seem to be related to serotonin's role in appetite, but other results suggest that rhythmic, repetitive movements of major muscle groups may be accompanied by increased serotonin system activity.

On the basis of this research, Dr. Jacobs in fact suggests that simple repetitive physical activities, such as riding a bicycle or jogging, might be beneficial for people suffering from depression. There are many reports of the antidepressant effects of running and other cardiovascular activities, as already mentioned, and his research points to a possible underlying mechanism. Exercise may directly stimulate serotonin system activity.

Obsessive-compulsive disorder (OCD), discussed in chapter 6, is a serotonin-associated disorder in which the anxious person feels compelled to repeat some action over and over again out of a fear of making a mistake. Often this is some repetitive ritual of checking, redoing, grooming, or cleaning. Dr. Jacobs has suggested that people with OCD may be calmed by their ritual because it serves to enhance serotonin activity. If so, they may be able to substitute other, more useful activities for the OCD ritual. A walk or other repetitive movements might save them from the potential harm of washing their hands over and over again until the skin roughens and cracks, or from the embarrassment of checking their work a hundred times, to the exasperation or confusion of their coworkers. He even speculates that obsessive thoughts, worries, fears, or fantasies that you can't stop going over and over might also have some serotonin-raising value that helps to explain why people experience them. Some fascinating new research provides a partial confirmation of Dr. Jacobs's theory.

You Can Change the Brain—New Evidence

OCD is a form of anxiety that is most often treated with serotonin-active drugs such as Prozac or Luvox, as detailed in chapter 6. A 1996 study by Jeffrey Schwartz and colleagues at the UCLA School of Medicine showed that physical activity and behavioral therapy actually resulted in changes in the brain that could be detected by PET scan. More recent studies have confirmed these results and shown, in addition, that the changes achieved with cognitive-behavioral therapy are comparable to those seen with antidepressant treatment—both for OCD and for other mood disorders. PET scanning provides images showing which areas of the brain are active at a given moment in time, based on detecting tiny differences in blood flow that indicate which areas are consuming more energy and doing more "brain work."

PET scans show that people with OCD have increased activity in three specific areas of the brain associated with alarm and vigilance. These areas seem to work together as a brain circuit that responds to danger, or the perception of danger. One area called the caudate nucleus, located deep within the brain, may have a gatekeeper influence on whether the "anxiety circuit" is activated. There is also evidence suggesting it is involved in the acquisition of habits and skills, and it has a wealth of connections with serotonin system brain centers that influence emotion and pain awareness. In people with OCD, serotonin-active drugs are known to reduce excess activity in this area, which is believed to excite the feelings of alarm and foreboding that drive OCD sufferers to redo and recheck everything. The PET scan findings show that the same brain changes can be achieved by nondrug therapies.

The approaches used included cognitive-behavioral therapy techniques, which involved teaching OCD sufferers how to control their obsessions and compulsions by relabeling their fears and impulses. Instead of giving in to an anxious need to wash the hands over and over again, they tell themselves, "I'm having a compulsion again. If I do something else, it'll go away." They would then pursue some enjoyable or productive activity for fifteen minutes, such as knitting or taking a walk. Carrying out this eight- to twelve-week program of rational self-talk and distracting physical activities was effective in changing how the brain functioned for six out of nine patients studied. Dr. Schwartz's research is generally focused on demonstrating that the mind *can* control the brain's chemistry. He hypothesized that the attention-diverting physical activity was the crucial step in altering the brain's activity patterns.

Did these changes result from altering or enhancing serotonin system functioning? Quite possibly, given what we know about OCD and serotonin. But the important point about this classic study—and confirmatory research that has followed it—is the encouragement it gives to those who want to bring their symptoms under control through lifestyle changes. It is reasonable to suppose, as a working hypothesis, that well-chosen physical activities can have a positive and lasting impact on controlling serotonin-related symptoms. The benefit is not only temporary or psychological—there are real biological changes in the brain.

What Kinds of Exercise or Activity?

The choice of an exercise program or activity depends on your health, stamina, and interests. You certainly want to choose something you enjoy that you can easily fit into your schedule and lifestyle. Many people who start a regular exercise program out of a sense of grim necessity—to trim down or to strengthen the heart and lungs—stay with it because of how much better they feel, mentally and physically, after each workout.

Start with the simplest activities and those requiring minimal or no investment. The basements and garages of America are full of dusty, unused exercise equipment. Bicycle if you already have a bicycle and enjoy it. Walking is another excellent choice, since all you need is a decent all-purpose athletic shoe or some other sturdy, well-cushioned shoe that provides good traction and support. If you play a sport but have not kept it up, you might enjoy finding a partner at your level and getting back into it. It is best to start with what you already know and already have. You will save both money and frustration by doing so! It is a good idea to have both indoor and outdoor activities you enjoy, so that you can take advantage of nice days but don't go without exercise when the weather is unfavorable.

The three key factors to consider, beyond preferences and equipment costs, have to do with deciding the intensity, frequency, and duration of exercise. The standard fitness-oriented recommendation sets the frequency and duration as at least twenty minutes three times a week. For pain and mood control, a weekly total of three hours is recommended. For full benefit in controlling your symptoms, you should find some form of physical activity you can do every day, preferably at the same time, even if it is only for ten minutes. Stretching exercises at the beginning or end of the day or a change in your daily routine that has you walking a few extra blocks are good choices. For example, if you work out of the home, you could park a little farther from your workplace or get off the bus a few blocks early.

Start with the Basics

When you wake up in the morning, do you yawn, stretch, and flex your back? If something takes you by surprise, do you take a big breath and then sigh? Well, those natural responses can be the basis for establishing your daily serotonin-enhancing exercises. You can start the day with stretching, flexing, and deep breathing. You can use these techniques to reduce pressure during the day. Or you can make them a "time to unwind" routine at the end of the workday, or in the evening after you put the kids to bed. Basic stretching and flexing exercises relax the body while lifting the mood. Here are a few easy-to-do exercises that provide the type of repetitive movements needed to boost serotonin activity.

Take a deep breath. Abdominal breathing relaxes the whole body and relieves stress and anxiety. Nothing could be simpler to do. Breathe in slowly, filling your lungs all the way with air. Hold for a second, exhale slowly. Repeat, slowly, five to ten times, while you focus on the sensation of the air flowing into your body and filling you up, from the abdomen to the neck.

Stretch and climb. Standing or sitting upright, reach your arms overhead, stretch and reach with each in turn, as though you were climbing a rope ladder. Repeat ten to twenty times.

Bend and bounce from the waist. While standing, bend over from the waist and reach for the floor with your arms, letting them dangle loosely. Bounce *gently* from the waist (don't strain or lurch!) while you relax your body. Repeat ten to twenty times.

Twist and turn. Stand with feet apart and each hand placed on its corresponding shoulder, elbows held level in the air. Turn side to side from the waist, turning your whole upper body, including your head and arms, with each gentle twist. As you turn to each side, extend your arm full length and then return your hand to your shoulder as you twist back. Repeat ten to twenty times.

Bend and bounce from the knees. Again standing with feet wide apart and pointed out, hold your back straight while you slowly bend your knees. Hold for one count, then slowly straighten your knees until you are almost standing, keeping your back straight as you do so. Repeat five to ten times. After you have built up some strength, bounce gently while you are in the knees-bent position.

Windmill swing. An exercise probably familiar to you from school days. Swing your arms in a full circle from the shoulders, first clockwise, then stop and swing counterclockwise. Start with just a few rotations and build up.

Leg lift. Standing, bend and lift the leg so that the thigh is parallel to the floor. Hold for one count, then let the leg drop to the floor. Alternating legs, repeat slowly as many times as you comfortably can. Keep your hand on a wall or other support for balance, if needed.

The finishing flourish. Do a more aerobic exercise that works the legs to finish up, such as jumping jacks, marching, or sprinting in place. You don't need to turn it into a full-scale workout, just a little burst of activity to quicken the heart for a few beats.

These exercises are for relaxing, stretching, and toning the body and shouldn't require sweating and straining. Don't make them tough or you won't want to do them.

Calming, Serotonin-Enhancing Activities

Formal exercise is not the only serotonin-enhancing activity. Any rhythmic, repetitive movement can increase serotonin system functioning—

such as those involved in many popular crafts and hobbies. The relaxing and soothing effects of knitting have more and more people, including men, taking up the craft. Knitting is easy and, once learned, can be done while watching TV or talking. Other hobbies, such as painting, sculpting, woodworking, and playing musical instruments, may yield similar results. The treatment program for OCD sufferers developed by Dr. Jeffrey Schwartz also provides partial support to the theory that the repetitive movements involved in these activities may have a real benefit in altering brain chemistry for the better.

If you still can't find an exercise or hobby that will interest you, Dr. Jacobs's research suggests that simply chewing gum might increase serotonin activity—both suppressing appetite and calming and lifting the mood. A snack of a crisp, chewy carbohydrate, such as an apple, celery, or carrots, might bring a double benefit in terms of increasing both serotonin activity and serotonin availability.

Aerobic Workouts for Maximum Results

Vigorous, aerobic exercise has long been known to elevate mood, and its effects last for several hours. Aerobic exercise is simply a level of physical activity that increases your rate of breathing for twenty minutes or longer. As the lungs and heart work to meet the physical demands, circulation improves, body temperature rises, warmed muscles begin to relax, and physical tension melts away. Serotonin is released in the brain, and endorphins are released in the body. The physical effort also distracts attention from any depressing or anxiety-producing preoccupations. If your problem is tension or anxiety, vigorous exercise effectively uses up the adrenaline and other hormones released in the fight-or-flight response to stress, which, after all, are meant to help you get moving to outrun any threats to your safety!

See your physician before attempting an aerobic exercise program, particularly if you are significantly overweight, have high blood pressure, kidney disease, heart disease, diabetes, or other serious medical problems—or if you are over forty and have not been exercising. Even if you are young and in good health, start with just a little more than your usual amount of exercise or exertion and build from there. All-out attempts will just leave you aching and limping, and very disinclined to try again.

For someone who has been mostly inactive, a twenty-minute walk on alternate days will probably provide a good starting point. As you exercise, monitor how you are doing. Breathing more quickly, sweating, and muscle warmth are good signs. If you feel faint, have sharp muscle pains, or have an irregular heartbeat or difficulty breathing, stop your workout. If you have any symptoms suggesting respiratory or heart problems, call your doctor at once. If you are comfortable during the workout and feel energized afterward, without any next-day muscle or joint pain, you are doing well. You can increase the pace or the distance on a weekly basis.

A walking speed of four miles per hour is a good goal for a reasonably fit person. If you would like to, you can try jogging after you have reached this pace. Begin by walking for a minute or two, until your muscles are warm and relaxed, then jog for one minute, followed by walking, then another minute of jogging and so on. When you can handle this pace well, after one to three walk-jog workouts, increase the jogging intervals to two minutes. Continue to add more minutes to the jogging until you are jogging the entire exercise time after an initial warm-up. If you do jog, you will need proper running shoes to avoid pain and injury. Also, a warm-up before jogging is advisable—either a walk or gentle stretching exercises to warm and loosen the Achilles tendon and calf and thigh muscles before the sudden stress of the run. Cool down after your run by walking slowly for a minimum of five minutes to maintain flexibility. Both walking and jogging can build bone strength and protect women against osteoporosis after menopause.

For low-cost indoor alternatives, check your local television listings to see if there is a half-hour aerobics program that you can work out to or record for later use. Alternatively, there are scores of exercise videotapes or DVDs available. Choose one that requires no equipment except perhaps for a step bench that you can make or buy cheaply.

The intensity of aerobic exercise can be estimated by how long it takes you to start huffing and puffing. If your workout has you panting after five to ten minutes, you can consider it vigorous; if you last fifteen or twenty minutes before your lungs begin to work harder, it is a moderate workout. Two other basic guidelines are the "talk" and "sweat" tests. If you are panting so hard that you cannot talk comfortably to an exercise buddy between breaths, you should slow down. On the other hand, if you do not need a shower after your workout, it may have been good exercise but would not be considered aerobic.

You can be more precise about measuring the aerobic value of your workout by monitoring your pulse rate before and after you exercise. Place the index and middle fingers of one hand gently but firmly on the inner wrist of the other, and locate the pulsing artery between the bone and the tendon. Count the pulses for ten seconds then multiply by six to get your pulse rate. Resting pulse rates are usually around 70 for men and 80 for women. The pulse should increase to about 120 to 130 for a healthy but nonathletic person doing moderate aerobic exercise. Many exercise machines will monitor your pulse rate while you work out, which is a nice advantage both for safety and for achieving your best workout level. Heart rate monitors are popular exercise accessories, but they are probably not worth the cost for recreational fitness activities. They are more useful for those who want to train competitively in their sport.

Your pulse rate is the same as your heart rate. As a very rough guide to your safe upper limit and your training capabilities, subtract your age from 220—the result approximates your maximum heart (pulse) rate. As you begin training, look first to increase your pulse rate by 50 percent over your resting pulse. Once you attain that goal, try for a 70 percent increase over the resting pulse at the height of your workout. That will give you the ideal cardiovascular benefits and will also leave you feeling your best. Whatever was bugging you before you began your workout will now be far from your serotonin-refreshed mind.

What Do You Like to Do?

Career counselors begin by taking stock of the individual's skills and interests. Then they offer a menu of matching jobs and professions. It is often an extremely helpful service to career changers and young job seekers because (a) we are often not aware of how many talents and abilities we have and (b) we are equally unaware of the number of career possibilities available to use those talents and abilities. You can identify your preferred serotonin-enhancing exercises, hobbies, and activities by using a similar history- and inventory-taking approach.

1. What are your strengths? Check any of the following for which you have average or above average capabilities for your age or among your circle of friends.

_____ Hand-eye coordination   _____ Arm strength
_____ Hand steadiness   _____ Leg strength
_____ Good vision   _____ Throwing and aiming ability
_____ Good hearing   _____ Stamina, endurance
_____ Good memory   _____ Speed, agility
_____ Physical flexibility   _____ Coordination

2. What sports, fitness activities, and hobbies have you participated in at some time in your life?

_____

_____

_____

_____

3. What potentially enjoyable sports, fitness activities, and hobbies would you be able to pursue right now?

_____

_____

_____

_____

4. What sports, fitness activities, and hobbies would you like to undertake in the future, if you further developed your fitness and skills?

_____

_____

_____

Serotonin-Enhancing Activities and Exercise

Repetitive Movement Activities

Sewing crafts

Knitting

Cooking

Musical instruments

Fishing

Painting

Woodworking

Jewelry-making and other crafts

Leisurely walking

Gardening

Moderate to Vigorous Aerobics

Brisk walking

Hiking, canoeing, rowing

Dancing, gymnastics

Swimming

Bicycling

Jogging, running

In-line skating

Cross-country skiing

Team sports—baseball, volleyball, basketball, field hockey, touch football

Aerobic fitness equipment— treadmills, stationary bikes, steppers, rowing and cross-country ski machines

Aerobic video workouts or classes

Racket sports—tennis, squash, racquetball, badminton, table tennis

Use Your Opportunities

It is undeniably hard to schedule regular exercise—our lives are too busy and our plans too easily disrupted. Since you can't always set aside time to exercise, why not look for opportunities to move around a bit more during your daily routine? For example, you might:

- Take the stairs rather than the elevator when you are just going one to three floors.
- Walk up and down escalators.
- Run errands on foot when you can; carrying packages is an extra benefit.
- Don't look for the parking space closest to the door. Head for the far end of the lot, where there are plenty of spaces. You'll get a little exercise, and no one will dent your car door!
- Park your car in a central location when you are in a shopping area. Walk between stores that are only a few blocks apart.
- Don't use labor-saving shortcuts; if your job and lifestyle are sedentary, do your physical chores and activities "the hard way."
- Counteract your own natural tendency to avoid moving. If you forget something you need or want, get up and go get it. Cultivate your absentmindedness. Get up once to get your book, another time to get a glass of juice or water.
- Remember to stretch, breathe, and flex whenever you are tired, anxious, or stressed.

Find a Way–Choose a Time

We know we should exercise more. We don't. The reasons for most people aren't hard to find. Exercise takes time. There isn't enough time. Or where you live and how you live limit the opportunities. If you commute between an industrial complex and a suburban development, you can't run errands on foot, so you lose a practical reason to take a walk. If you live in the north, cold weather and bad weather may keep you indoors most of the winter, so walking, running, and bicycling are less appealing. And, besides, there always seem to be more reasons *not* to exercise, more important priorities for limited leisure time and breaks.

Yet a few well-chosen minutes of exercise or physical activity can give you the energy and mood lift to make better use of the rest of your day either for work or play. The half hour or hour invested in exercise will yield a handsome time dividend by improving daytime alertness and the quality of your sleep. If you have impulse control problems, such as eating, drinking, or overspending, exercise can be one of the best serotonin-enhancing diversions available. There is always a way to add exercise to your life.

As you begin to consider your exercise options, you may find it much easier to get motivated if you focus on a simple, positive goal: feeling better. You may be very focused on losing weight, and view exercise as an effective, but unpleasant and difficult means to accomplish that goal. Try to put your weight-loss or body image issues out of your mind as you begin to choose your exercise program. If you select a negative goal ("I look awful—I have to get more exercise"), you are more likely to feel defeated or discouraged when you don't instantly drop pounds.

Instead, pay attention to the mood and energy reward you experience after your exercise. Whether it's a high-energy aerobics class in the morning or a relaxing half-mile walk at lunchtime or around dinnertime, you will get a boost that you may have been seeking—but not getting—from food. If you pay attention to the positive feelings generated by exercise, you will find it much easier to get over the reluctance and inertia most people feel about taking on health and fitness programs that they view as "something I'm supposed to do (but don't really want to)."

A little effort and imagination can build other incentives into regular exercise. Find a friend—a neighbor at home or a coworker during the week—who can join you in a walk or some other exercise like bicycling or swimming. Turning exercise into a social event makes it much more enjoyable, and also harder to neglect or back out of. Keeping a simple calendar of your exercise also helps as a motivator. If you add stats to this record, such as how far, how fast, or how long, you can have the pleasure of competing against yourself and seeing your progress.

There are always opportunities for just a little exercise, and, as we noted, a little may nonetheless achieve a significant serotonin-enhancing effect. If you work at a desk and have limited opportunities to get out and about, use your breaks to do deep breathing and relaxation exercises. If you have the opportunity, take a walk or run errands on foot when a craving strikes. If cigarette smokers are motivated by their habit to stand outside in the coldest and wettest weather, surely you can put on a coat and walk around the block while on your break. Exercise is one of the best mood-stimulants and appetite-suppressants available—much better than the ones that come in bottles of pills!

11

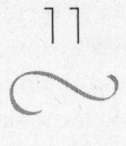

Targeting Your
Serotonin Symptoms

As we have seen, the manifestations of reduced serotonin functioning can take many different forms, but usually include low mood, low energy, and low motivation, often accompanied by poor control over eating, drinking, or other problem behaviors. These problems might strike at specific times of the year, month, or day. You may have up and down swings that last a few hours or a few days. Whatever the pattern and the problem, adopting a serotonin-friendly lifestyle will produce real benefits for most people with mild to moderate symptoms. However, we aren't "just chemicals" and we certainly aren't just one chemical. If you have specific symptoms that are more severe or long-term, they may not respond fully to improved nutrition and exercise alone. For example, if you have been living with anxiety, depression, or chronic pain for a long time, if it has become your life—you may need more specific interventions to help you. Or if you have low self-esteem and are very self-critical, the boost you get from better food and activity will be temporary—not powerful enough to offset your long-established habits of thinking and feeling about yourself. This chapter will offer you additional help and guidance by summarizing in simplified form some of the behavioral (nondrug) strategies health professionals offer for dealing with problems with appetite and impulse control, poor sleep, low or anxious mood, and migraine and other chronic headaches.

Do behavioral strategies and interventions work by raising brain serotonin levels or by stimulating the serotonin system into higher levels of activity? On a theoretical level, any activity, mental or physical, that improves mood, sleep, and appetite control can be assumed to be acting on the serotonin system in some way. On a practical level, these strategies work for those who make the commitment and the effort to try, and that's the basis for recommending them. Positive self-talk and cognitive therapy strategies can have real, cumulative effects on the brain's mood chemistry, as shown by the PET scan research briefly described in chapter 10. Others are simply helpful hints and tried-and-true wisdom from fellow sufferers.

Positive Self-Talk for Better Mood Control

Even when negative moods are not the primary serotonin-related symptom, negative mood can be a significant accompanying problem. For this reason, anything you can do to improve your mood or sustain a positive mood will help with other serotonin-related symptoms.

You can influence your mood biochemistry not only by your activities and foods but also by your thoughts and your frame of mind. Remember the placebo effect discussed in chapter 4. Hope and determination are powerful medicine, with no negative side effects.

Don't respond to your anxious or low feelings or your lack of energy and interest with an attitude of passive acceptance—talk back to them! While you certainly might have a reason to feel low (work pressures, a fight with your spouse, family worries, etc.), you may feel worse because of some serotonin system deficiency you can detect and correct. When a negative mood strikes, probe and question it. Ask yourself if your feelings are really in proportion to the event or problem that seemed to trigger them. If not, you can say to yourself, "There's nothing really all that wrong. My mood is a symptom. It doesn't mean anything and I shouldn't give in to it. I can do a little deep breathing, take a walk, have a pasta salad for lunch, or a piece of fruit for a snack. I'll feel better if I do, and then I'll be more my normal self."

A negative mood usually brings with it negative thoughts. When your mood chemistry shifts you down, you begin to brood about every stupid thing you ever did, every major disappointment you ever experienced, every terrible catastrophe that might happen to you, and all the things you pick on about yourself as inferior, dumb, ugly, or unlovable. Suddenly, you are your own worst enemy! Because mood shifts can sneak up on us, we tend to think that the negative thoughts come first. In fact, it's the other way around. First the chemistry changes, and then come the negative, anxious, self-critical ideas. A change in brain chemistry, primarily a drop in serotonin functioning, is making you focus on all the bad stuff in your life and forget the good.

When a negative mood strikes, imagine that the self-condemnation and self-criticism taking place in your head is actually being debated in a courtroom. The prosecutor is relentlessly detailing everything that is wrong with you and your life. Now it is the defense attorney's turn—what do you have to say on behalf of the defendant? Rather than pleading guilty as charged, you jump to your own defense like a good lawyer, answering every charge point by point.

"No, it is not true that I will lose my job because of the mistake I made last week; in fact, I have one of the best performance records in the company."

"No, it is not true that I am hideously fat and my thighs are gigantic sausages. I'm a few pounds overweight, like almost everybody I know, and I ate a few cookies. Is that a crime? I can't expect to be perfect and to control my eating every single moment of every day.

I've been getting more exercise, and I'm looking and feeling pretty good."

This kind of positive self-talk is the essence of cognitive therapy, which involves learning to dismiss negative thinking that is exaggerated and illogical by countering it with more moderate, reasonable, and positive views. If you have persistent, depressed, or anxious thoughts, you might find it helpful to work through your negativity with pen and paper, or computer and keyboard. Sometimes writing down your bad feelings about yourself can help you be more objective and better able to counter the bad with the good.

If you refuse to believe in your negative mood, if you see it as a symptom that's going to go away, not much different from a stomachache or a bruised shin, then it will be much less overwhelming—more like the imaginary bogeymen that were once hiding under your bed when you were very small and afraid of loneliness and the unknown, as we all still are.

Punch Out PMS

Until we are certain of the underlying causes and mechanism of premenstrual syndrome, we can't really speak with confidence about preventing its more severe symptoms. Many women, however, only experience slight premenstrual changes, with temporary bloating and weight gain. Others may have to look at the calendar to know their period is about due. Is this luck of the genes or lifestyle? No one can say for sure. But studies have shown that improving nutrition and exercising regularly provide significant benefits. Women prone to PMS tend to overconsume salt, sugar, and animal fat. Changing to a low-sugar, low-animal fat, high-carbohydrate diet has produced good results for some, quite possibly due to effects on the serotonin system. Aerobic exercise (in one study, a running program averaging 1.5 miles per day) has been shown to have benefits on a wide range of PMS symptoms, from breast tenderness to irritable mood. It's not clear whether these good results are specific to PMS symptoms or reflect the general improvement in mood and pain tolerance that regular exercise provides.

Control Your PMS

- Follow a low sodium diet to reduce or eliminate edema (bloating).
- Cut back on fat and meat—increase fruit, vegetable, water, and grains in your diet.
- Fight food cravings, especially for high-salt, high-fat, and high-sugar foods.
- Exercise regularly, with special attention to the PMS days and the week preceding them.
- Keep a journal of your symptoms to identify patterns and successful prevention strategies.
- Consider vitamin supplementation (particularly B complex and iron) if you are not getting good results from improved nutrition.

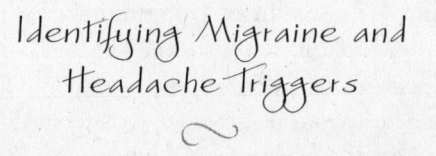

Identifying Migraine and Headache Triggers

Chronic headaches cannot be cured but they can often be avoided. Common triggers for many headaches include stress (the big one), muscle tension, too much or too little sleep, skipped meals, eyestrain, excessive glare, and, of course, excessive alcohol. If your work and hobbies involve close work, including reading, writing, keyboarding, and working at a computer monitor, try to limit the strain on your eyes. Look up frequently, focusing for a moment of relaxation on some object in the distance, or at least a few feet away. Keep computer monitors clean, and get an antiglare screen if you think it would help. If you have frequent, stress-related headaches or weekend and vacation letdown headaches, practice relaxation techniques several times daily, such as abdominal breathing and the stretch-and-relax exercises described in chapter 10. Some additional tension-releasing exercises are described in this chapter.

Hundreds of migraine triggers have been reported, although an individual migraine sufferer may have only a few significant ones. Unavoidable ones include weather and barometric pressure, which no one can do anything about. Almost unavoidable ones include hormones—for women migraines are often timed with the menstrual cycle. Bright, flickering, or flashing lights can bring on migraines for many sufferers, as can sharp, rhythmic, or loud noises. Intense penetrating odors, from perfume to paint, can trigger an attack, and so can steam or poor ventilation, as in a stuffy office building. Migraine sufferers are often more susceptible to motion sickness and some will get a migraine from roller-coaster rides and even from rocking chairs! It's as though the migraine sufferer's nervous system is acutely sensitive to any sensory overload or excess stimulation.

Dietary triggers can be the most important to identify, since they can be more easily controlled than many of the environmental factors. The list of possible dietary factors is long, and most migraine sufferers will be vulnerable to just a few of them. Unfortunately, for people who rely heavily on prepared supermarket foods and fast food, it can be just about impossible to decide which ingredient out of dozens is the culprit. However, doing this detective work can offer you tremendous benefit in reducing your migraine frequency. A roundup of the usual suspects includes:

- Foods containing MSG (monosodium glutamate)—almost any prepared food, literally from soups to seasoned nuts, can contain MSG; it is often listed simply as "natural flavor," so you cannot rely on label reading to avoid it
- Foods containing high amounts of tyramine—including red wine and beer, aged cheeses, smoked meats, smoked fish, pickled herring, sour cream, yogurt, and yeast extracts

- Foods containing nitrites—including bacon, packaged lunch meats, hot dogs, ham, sausage, and cold cuts
- Some types of beans, including lima, fava, and Chinese pea pods and sugar snap bean pods
- Foods containing high amounts of refined sugar or corn syrup
- The artificial sweetener aspartame (NutraSweet, Equal)
- Large quantities of citrus fruits
- Smoked and pickled foods
- Pork, liver, sweetbreads, and other organ meats
- Chocolate (sorry!)
- Alcohol, even in amounts too small to trigger a hangover headache
- Caffeine, which can either trigger or treat headaches, somewhat unpredictably
- Dietary deficiencies, particularly of B-complex vitamins

Tyramine is an amino acid, a necessary building block of protein, but large quantities of it in a meal can apparently trigger changes in blood vessels that result in migraine. No research has yet documented an effect of MSG on the brain and nervous system, yet many headache experts, like headache sufferers, are convinced that it is a potent trigger for approximately one-third of all migraine sufferers. If you do have a vulnerability to MSG, it is increasingly difficult to avoid. Americans consume about one-third of a pound of MSG annually, and it is found very widely in convenience food, whether canned, frozen, or packaged. Virtually the only way to avoid it is to rely on fresh foods—a great overall health strategy, but difficult for people who do not always have the time to prepare their own meals. If your migraines are frequent and severe, you may well be motivated to try. For some canned foods, such as tuna or beans, you may find that rinsing the food in a strainer is somewhat effective for flushing out the MSG as well as any other added sodium.

You should not assume that any of these foods trigger your migraines until you have observed and documented a clear connection. Suppose you get a horrible migraine after you binge on chocolate, following an argument with your boyfriend, on an overcast and stormy day, about three days before your period is due? That's four possible triggers right there. Which one is responsible?

There are two ways to find out. If your migraines are truly terrible, you may want to try a thirty-day elimination diet. Avoid every known migraine trigger, restricting your food and beverage intake to fresh and homemade foods, where you have complete control over the ingredients. There are plenty of simple meals based on pasta, lean meats, poultry, fresh fish, and rice to choose from. Most of the recommendations in chapter 10 are appropriate for a migraine sufferer's trigger-avoiding diet.

With the elimination diet, you want to track any migraines you suffer during the thirty days and spot any connections with daily stress, irregular eating or sleeping, menstrual cycle, weather, and other environmental triggers. Keep a careful daily record, as described in chapter 12, of all your headaches and any other serotonin-related symptoms such as mood. Then, in the following month, add one suspected food back to your diet at a time. Consume it on three separate occasions in significant quantities before you decide it is safe to add back to your diet. Then move on to test another potential trigger. This approach to identifying and eliminating dietary triggers takes more effort and commitment, but can yield big benefits in long-term pain prevention. And it is certainly preferable to eliminating whole categories of food from your diet on suspicion only! One recent study examined how dietary restrictions and avoidance of environmental triggers might benefit migraine sufferers. The researchers documented a 50 percent decline in migraine frequency, with significant reductions in headache duration and severity among the study's participants.

For people with less frequent migraines, keeping a daily Food-Mood-Activity Journal, as described in chapter 12, will provide essential leads for identifying migraine triggers. You will want to expand your journal to include information on other possible headache triggers, as well as recording the positive and negative influences of your eating and activities on your mood and pain problem.

Many migraine sufferers experience food cravings before or around the time of their headache attacks—perhaps because of serotonin system changes that include effects on appetite, impulse, pain, and blood vessels in the brain. If you have both food cravings and headaches as PMS symptoms or at times of stress, try satisfying your craving with a trigger-free complex carbohydrate, such as noncitrus fruits, vegetables, or crackers. See if you can reduce the intensity and frequency of the headaches by controlling your snacking at headache-prone times. Much clinical experience suggests that premigraine food cravings might actually be migraine triggers.

Quick Steps to Headache Prevention

- Limit caffeine intake, including coffee, tea, and caffeinated soft drinks.
- Keep a headache journal to identify food triggers and patterns.
- Avoid convenience foods if you have MSG sensitivity.
- Don't give in to food cravings that strike at headache-prone times.
- Build up to three hours a week of aerobic exercise—more if you can.

Mind over Stomach: Managing IBS

- Exercise is a universally effective stress reducer that may offer specific benefits for IBS with either diarrhea or constipation. Slow, rhythmic relaxing exercise can ease abdominal cramping. A stationary bike (check garage sales and thrift stores for bargains) would be a good choice here. Regular daily or near-daily exercise is very helpful for avoiding constipation. (Move it to move it!)
- Don't eat on the run, or while stressed or distracted. Try to make snacks and mealtimes an occasion for relaxing and enjoying. Eat smaller meals more frequently if large portions tend to bring on

cramping. Close your eyes, take a few deep breaths, and calm yourself before eating *anything*. Reserve a few minutes for sitting quietly after you eat, before resuming stressful or hectic activities.

- Consider whether high-fat foods may be a problem for you. Fat digestion requires a special metabolic process that proceeds more slowly than digestion of protein, starch, and sugar. A sudden increase in fat intake—a big meal with a rich dessert, or a series of such meals—can result in queasiness, followed by either constipation or diarrhea, or one followed by the other. Some people may be habitually consuming more fat than their bodies can process, producing recurrent bouts of those all-too-familiar, agonizing cramps. Use a Food–Mood–Activity Journal to assess whether too much fat or particular high-fat foods (dairy foods or fatty meats like cold cuts) may be contributing to your symptoms.

- For IBS with diarrhea, avoid foods containing the sugar substitute sorbitol or high levels of fructose sugar, since these are poorly absorbed in the gastrointestinal tract. Keep a Food–Mood–Activity Journal (as explained in chapter 12) to monitor for possible food allergies (dairy, wheat, high-fat foods) or for negative effects of high-fiber foods. All those officially good-for-you foods like raw vegetables, unpeeled fruit, and whole-grain bread may be just too much for a sensitive digestive tract to process. If you currently follow a rigorously healthy, whole food–based diet, try substituting more cooked vegetables for all those salads; peel raw produce and chew it thoroughly to break down the fiber. You never know—it might help!

- For IBS with constipation, review your diet to see if you are getting enough fiber from relatively unprocessed foods like whole wheat and other grains, vegetables, and fruit. Use a Food–Mood–Symptom Journal to track whether high-fat foods might be bringing on symptoms. If you have been relying too heavily on refined and processed foods, try avoiding high-fat foods and adding more fiber *gradually* to your diet, along with adequate fluids, preferably water. Too much fiber all at once can bring on more bloating and gassiness. If you tend to be very sensitive to fiber, then try small servings. For example, have pasta as a side dish, not the main course; see if you do better with fruits and vegetables when they are peeled and well cooked rather than raw.

Beating Insomnia

If you are prone to insomnia, you will want to pay special attention to how foods affect you. Alcohol will put people to sleep, but they generally sleep badly, often awakening in the middle of the night. If you are hungry before bed and feel food might help you relax, a fat-containing carbohydrate snack would be a good choice, such as a few crackers with peanut butter or cheese. You should avoid going to bed with a too-full stomach. The intestinal "brain" usually goes into deep-wave sleep along with the brain; it cannot do so if a large meal or snack is still being digested. Many people will sleep poorly and suffer from heartburn from eating too much too late at night.

As chapter 3 explained, melatonin production normally gears up as soon as the lights are out. It stops abruptly when light strikes the retina of the eye. If your insomnia is related to a serotonin-melatonin problem, you will want to make sure that you keep your bedroom absolutely dark, with drapes or blinds completely blocking out any street light. If you get up during the night to use the bathroom, don't flip on the light, but instead have a night light in your bathroom that will provide adequate but minimal illumination. So long as dangling cords, loose rugs, and other hazards are removed, you should be able to navigate a familiar path in your own home without any light at all.

If you do wake up during the night and cannot get back to sleep, it is best to get up. Keeping room lights as dim as possible, you can try having a small low-sugar snack, listening to soft music, or reading a not-too-exciting book, preferably using a not-too-bright task light for illumination. Any calming repetitive movement, such as knitting or rocking yourself, may also be a wonderful sedative to get you ready to go back to bed. After a night of unsatisfactory sleeping, consider how your day's activities might have affected you. Did you have too much caffeine or alcohol? Did you get too little exercise? Did you try to go to sleep too soon after work, household clean-up chores, or struggling to get your children put to bed, without allowing yourself any time to unwind? Try to spot any daytime problems that may have contributed to your bad night and avoid them in the future.

Sleep-Tight Tips

- Exercise in the late afternoon or early evening can help relax and tire the body for quiet evening hobbies, followed by bedtime; however don't try to go to bed too soon after stimulating aerobic exercise.
- Avoid caffeine after 3 P.M., including teas and caffeinated sodas.
- Confine your alcohol consumption to one or two servings with dinner. Don't drink late in the evening.
- Limit fluid intake after 8 P.M. If your dinner makes you thirsty, you probably need to cut back on your salt intake.
- Keep the last hour or two of the evening free for relaxing and fun. Don't let work or household chores deprive you of this needed unwind time.
- If you were depending on alcohol to help you relax, try deep breathing and relaxation exercises (described later in this chapter) in the last hour of the evening.
- You can try a small late-night snack, such as crackers with or without cheese; hot herbal tea might help, too.
- Don't sleep late to make up for a bad night. Getting up at your regular time—and getting an early dose of bright morning light—will help reset your body's clock so that the next night's sleep will be better. In fact, sleep restriction is a good short-term treatment for both insomnia and depression.

- Keep regular hours, not just during the week but on the weekends too. If your serotonin-melatonin clock is easily thrown out of sync by a late night out, a regular schedule can be very important to feeling better as well as sleeping better. It may be hard to leave at ten or eleven when you know your friends are going to party well past midnight. But the spin-off benefit is that your weekend mornings can be devoted to doing something much more enjoyable than pulling the covers over your head!

- If you have night owl insomnia and are generally sedentary, getting some early A.M. outdoor exercise, such as a half-hour walk on your way to work, can help in resetting the body's clock for a more reasonable bedtime. In the evening, keep overhead lights dimmed or turned off. Use task lighting, such as a reading lamp, for hobbies, reading, deskwork, and other interests.

- For night-shift workers, good strategies to help make day of night and night of day include bright lights in the workplace, wraparound sunglasses for the commute home, then going directly to a fully darkened bedroom for relaxation and sleep. If you come home just as your family is getting up, let them understand that you need things quiet so you can catch up with your sleep. You can catch up with their lives at the end of the day.

People with irregular sleep often acquire a dependence on caffeine, alcohol, and sedatives that can make their sleep problems much worse. If you are overusing caffeine as your daytime stimulant and alcohol as your nighttime relaxant, it may seem terribly difficult to cut back—until you see how great the benefit can be. Adapt your Food-Mood-Activity Journal (see chapter 12) to include detailed information on how you sleep—how long it takes you to fall asleep (approximately), if you get up in the night to empty your bladder, and how long it takes you to fall back asleep if you do wake up during the night. Make yourself try every one of the suggestions for general insomnia given above, at least once, and document the impact on your sleep.

Getting a Grip on Anxiety

Positive self-talk and other cognitive therapy techniques can be directed to defeating obsessive worries and fears. Write down your worries and argue back. Instead of ruminating on what-if, get out a sheet of paper. Draw a line down the middle of it. On the left side, write down what's bothering you. On the right, talk back to your anxiety. Say why it's probably going to be okay. For example:

It's one o'clock in the morning! She promised to be back by eleven, and she hasn't called. I know something's happened . . . a car accident . . . she's lying hurt somewhere.

My daughter's growing up—she'll be in college next year. Some of her friends are already on their own. She's tired of her parents treating her like a kid. She's having fun and lost track of the time. She won't call because my worrying annoys her and she thinks her friends will make fun of her for "having a curfew."

OR:

I messed up, big time. I'm going to lose my job. We need my income—how are we going to pay the bills?

Okay, I made a mistake. But I've had a really good track record and a lot of accomplishments. So-and-so's basically incompetent and they've never fired him. And then there's what's-his-name—he lost a major account two years ago and he's still with the company.

Many people who have interpreted their physical anxiety symptoms as a sign they are seriously ill have limited their exercise, yet vigorous exercise is an enormous help in releasing anxiety. You should certainly be evaluated by your doctor before beginning an exercise program if you have any symptoms suggesting a possible heart or lung abnormality. If your health permits, exercise can be one of the best nondrug treatments for anxiety. A vigorous aerobic workout puts the fight-or-flight response of anxiety to good use. Sometimes anxiety will intensify for the first few minutes of an aerobic workout, and then fade as the muscles warm and relax. You will feel physically relaxed afterward, with the tension released from your body and mind. These antianxiety effects of exercise will last for about four hours for most people. You may still have significant problems you need to solve, but the painful anxiety that limits your ability to focus and take action will be greatly diminished.

If your health doesn't allow you to exercise vigorously, or you just can't face it right now, even swinging your arms or lying on your back and "bicycling" with your legs in the air can help you release muscular tension. Other calming activities include relaxation exercises and deep abdominal breathing (covered in chapter 10).

If your problem is not chronic worry but performance or social anxiety or a phobia of some sort, the best approach, and the one used by experts, is to confront the fear step-by-step. For example, if you find it hard to socialize with new people, accept one of those invitations you usually reject, and set a goal to talk to one new person. You would be well advised not to target the most attractive person in the room, and instead begin by choosing people who will not interpret your friendliness as sexual interest. Realize that most people have some level of discomfort, and your courage and friendliness will probably be appreciated. Cleverness and originality are not required, "Great appetizers, aren't they?" will do just fine, or even a more direct, "Hi, my name's _____. I'm one of _____'s friends from high school."

If public speaking is painful for you, try practicing on family members, or even perfect strangers! Your main concern may be that you can't bring yourself to ask questions at meetings or seminars, or you can't comfortably make the presentations you need to do in order to advance in your job. To loosen up and gain experience, you can experiment with speaking up in unstressful situations. For example, if you're standing in a line or waiting for a late train, say something to the people standing near you—a gripe about the wait, or better yet a joke about it. If you are generally shy with strangers, try making friendly small talk with checkout clerks, bank tellers, and other service industry professionals. All but the most bored and grumpy will tend to respond with appreciation at being treated like people rather than automatons. When you can comfortably start and lead a conversation with strangers, you will gradually gain the poise to speak in more stressful or intimidating settings.

Since so many of the troubling symptoms of anxiety are physical, both relaxation techniques and aerobic exercise may help you with the physical manifestations of your nervousness by improving your cardiovascular tone and your self-control.

No Need for Alarm: How to Curb Anxiety

- Avoid caffeine—coffee, tea, and caffeinated soft drinks.
- Use aerobic exercise to prevent or control anxious preoccupations—as often and vigorous as health and stamina allow.
- Practice relaxation exercises when stressed or worried.
- Distract yourself from obsessions and compulsions with relaxing physical activities—walks, hobbies, or arts and crafts.
- Practice cognitive therapy techniques to control worrying.

Exercise, Mental Focus, and Anxiety

There is yet another aspect to serotonin's relationship to physical activity. As mentioned in chapter 2, serotonin activity is suppressed in animals when they freeze to pay attention to a sudden sound or sight. Serotonin is believed to play a role in switching the nervous system between movement and attention to sensory information. If this basic function holds true for humans, as it almost surely does, it indicates that serotonin activity drops when some sight or sound gets your attention. People in a state of anxiety are readily characterized as nervous or jumpy. They are hyperalert to sudden noises, are easily startled, and tend to scan their surroundings visually more than other people, as though they were always on the lookout for danger. It may be that this jumpy, all-ears, all-eyes state acts to depress serotonin activity. If so, we make ourselves feel worse by giving in to the panicked all-systems alert state. If you find yourself worrying obsessively, try doing some simple repetitive exercises (see chapter 10 for suggestions) in a quiet location, where you can focus on a pleasant view or a picture on a wall.

The calming and refreshing effects of yoga and of deep breathing and relaxation exercises may be related to this phenomenon. These activities all involve the combination of movement with visualizing, mental focusing, and meditation techniques that turn attention inward, away from distracting stimuli in the environment. Interestingly, meditation can calm some anxious people while others will sometimes experience a sudden onset of panic symptoms a few minutes into their meditation. Perhaps classical meditation techniques that require the individual to hold perfectly still act to lower serotonin activity to a level that is counterproductive for some individuals. Or it may be that the "turn inward" technique invites the anxious person to focus on physical symptoms such as heartbeat.

If you are troubled by anxiety, a combination of exercise and meditation may be very beneficial. If you feel yourself becoming anxious or preoccupied with worries at a time when it is not possible to stop what you are doing for extended exercise, develop a simple one-minute ritual to calm yourself down. Close your eyes, take a few slow, deep abdominal breaths, exhaling slowly, and tell yourself, "It's okay, these are just my symptoms. Nothing is really wrong."

Another exercise for relieving anxiety, tension, and anger involves tensing and relaxing your muscle groups, one at a time. Working from the ground up, curl your toes tightly, then release and relax. Flex (bend) your feet up so that the muscles of your calf are tense, then relax and extend the foot. Stretch and tighten your legs, so the muscles are tense, then flex and relax. Next, tighten your stomach, then release. Make a fist with each hand and then shake your fingers and wrist loose. Flex your biceps and relax. Finally, squeeze your face into a grimace, then release. Visualizing and thinking "The tension is going into my foot (leg, stomach, etc.)—now it's gone" can also help you focus on chasing the tension out of your body and mind.

Appetite and Impulse Control

Bingeing, craving, and other impulse control problems often stem from underlying problems with negative mood—stress, tension, disappointment, anxiety, or just a general feeling of being deprived, misused, neglected, or overburdened. If you are normally cheerful and energetic, this description may not seem to match your personality. Yet you may be medicating your stress with food so automatically that you are not aware of the feelings that drive you to reach for a fattening snack or—for that matter—an extravagant purchase or a drink. Consider times when you, like everyone else, eat on the run because of a hectic schedule. Do you cram more food into your mouth more quickly than you normally would if you were able to sit down and enjoy your meal?

Whenever possible, use your lunch hour and breaks to get a little exercise, if only by stretching and walking around a little. If you do have an hour to yourself at midday, try to devote thirty or forty-five minutes to walking. If you are a compulsive shopper, stay clear of the stores; tell yourself you must keep your feet in motion. You can come back at the end of the workday to check out any appealing sales or window displays. Reserve as much time as you need to eat comfortably, without rushing, before going back to work. If you like to have a goal, you can take care of a necessary errand or two, unless you find you are spending too much time waiting in noon-hour lines at the bank or the store. Whether your walk is in the middle of a busy downtown, a park, or your own neighborhood, you will find that both the diversion and the exercise will send you back to your tasks feeling relaxed and restored.

Dieting: Don't Do It!

Even if bingeing and food cravings have resulted in the gain of extra pounds you are anxious to lose, formal, restrictive diets should be avoided. As explained in chapter 7, the deprivation and the potential nutritional imbalances that result from dieting will invariably trigger hard-to-control cravings and possibly increased bingeing, particularly if dieting lowers your serotonin supply. Several studies have reported that low-calorie dieting reduces circulating tryptophan levels, resulting in lower availability to the brain and reduced serotonin production. Interestingly, this effect was greater in women than in men. In reviewing the evidence, Howard Steiger, among others, has suggested that dieting might be a *cause* of bulimia in women.

Diets are not only difficult, but may be literally depressing for some women. One study by Oxford researcher Philip Cowen and colleagues compared the mood and serotonin effects of a three-week crash diet (1,000 calories a day) in two groups of women—those with a history of major depression and those without. Those with a history of depression showed an impaired ability to adapt brain serotonin system functioning to a lower availability of tryptophan. The researchers concluded that:

- Women with a vulnerability to major depression have an impaired regulation of brain serotonin function during a weight reduction diet.
- This impairment may predispose them to a return of low-mood symptoms during dieting.

This negative effect of dieting seems strongest in depression-prone women who are significantly overweight or who gained weight during their depression. While a slight reduction in calories might be neutral or beneficial, it would be very important to track mood during any attempts at dieting. *Lowered serotonin availability may be the invisible string producing the yo-yo effect of repeated failed diets.*

If you follow the healthy carbohydrate guidelines and sample menu suggestions given in chapter 9, you will have a gradual reduction in binge-ing and in weight. Do not set your sights on becoming thin. If you have been overweight for much of your adult life and have gone through re-peated episodes of yo-yo dieting, a reasonable and more attainable goal is preventing further weight gain, with perhaps a gradual decline of a pound a month. If you are overweight and have a history of alternating bingeing and dieting, you may have convinced yourself that your self-esteem and future happiness depend on losing weight. Try to lose that idea. *Your diet-ing may be a major factor in your mood and eating problems.* Remember: No one overeats because they are happy. If you can choose a lifestyle that lifts your mood, over the long term your weight will go down.

One study compared the long-term weight loss experienced by three groups of overweight volunteers. The first group was put on a pro-gram of dieting only, the second group followed a program of exercise only without dieting, and the third group was given a program that com-bined dieting with exercise. Would you like to guess which group suc-ceeded in both losing weight and keeping it off? Surprisingly, the volunteers who exercised only, without dieting, had the best results. They lost fewer pounds but they didn't gain them back again, unlike the di-eters. Based on their interviews with the study participants, the re-searchers concluded that those who both dieted and exercised evidently found the combination so restrictive and burdensome that they were not able to keep to the program after the initial rapid weight loss. They gained it all back. In contrast, those who exercised did not feel deprived of the pleasure food provides. They came to enjoy exercise for the mood and energy lift it gives, and so they were able to make it a permanent part of their lifestyle.

Exercise, but don't deprive yourself of the pleasure of food. Keep your meals and snacks pleasant and satisfying by giving them your full attention. If you do eat at your desk, don't try to work, read the newspaper, or surf the Web simultaneously. Get the maximum enjoyment from what you eat by savoring each bite, holding it in your mouth, and enjoying the flavors. Stay away from fake foods, such as low-fat cheeses and sugar-free desserts. Often these low-calorie artificial contrivances of the processed food industry only remind you of what you are missing. Unless eating truly gives you the pleasure you seek, negative feelings may drive you to eat again an hour or two later, out of dissatisfaction rather than real appetite.

Try to select foods that cannot be wolfed down in a few bites, such as salads and fruit or relatively chewy breads. Since spaghetti is notoriously hard to balance gracefully on a fork, it is a good complex carbohydrate to eat socially, where you must mind your table manners! If you like Asian food, use chopsticks. You will impress everyone with your sophistication while controlling your appetite better. If you have a sandwich for lunch, remind yourself to put the sandwich down after each bite.

A key strategy for controlling impulses such as excessive snacking, drinking, or out-of-control spending is something we all know how to do—procrastinate! When a strong, hard-to-suppress urge to eat or drink comes over you, check the time. Tell yourself that you will give in to the urge in one hour, if you haven't changed your mind in the interim. Use that hour for serotonin-enhancing activities and exercises if you can, such as a walk or a hobby or other activity that involves relaxing, repetitive movements. If work and other responsibilities limit your freedom during that hour, give your mouth and your appetite a substitute pleasure. Chew gum or have a piece of fruit or a complex carbohydrate such as bread or a not-too-sweet muffin. If your impulse problem is alcohol, serotonin-enhancing exercise is the recommended solution, followed, if you like, by a nonalcoholic beer or spicy Bloody Mary mix that you can sip slowly.

If you are a compulsive shopper, tell yourself that you must wait a minimum of twenty-four hours, better yet three days, before buying that got-to-have-it item. Don't sell yourself on it with the idea that it will be gone if you wait. Maybe it will, but in these days of mass production, chain stores, and online outlets, it can be reordered or found somewhere else. If your shopping is influenced by sales, try to stay away from them, or go with the firm intention of purchasing only those things you had already decided you needed and wanted. If you see something else that tempts you, make yourself hold out for the whole three days. It may be the same price or marked even lower if and when you go back to get it. You can learn to play sales like playing the stock market. An astute shopper will follow a hunch that the price will drop even lower. The times you guess right and wait will provide you with more pleasure than you get from grabbing the goods and running to the cash register.

Basically, you tell your impulse, "If I really love you, I'll wait for you." If the impulse goes away before the time is up, then it was just a passing infatuation, not the real thing.

The 3 Ds of Impulse Control

- **D**elay. Tell yourself you'll wait an hour to have that snack, or a day to make that purchase.
- **D**istract yourself. Take a walk, do an errand, have a healthy serotonin-enhancing snack.
- **D**on't deprive yourself. Diets and other forms of self-denial don't help control serotonin-deficient impulses but will only make them worse.

What about Ordinary Overeating?

Like birds or grazing antelopes, sometimes it seems as if we were designed by nature to spend all our time eating. It is so much easier to eat than to resist eating when food is right in front of us—as it always is. What do you do to control normal urges to polish off the ice cream, the cookies, or the chips?

The first is simply to keep tempting ready-made foods out of your house. If you have growing kids, you may feel you need to keep cookies and other treats on hand for them. But what is bad for you is not all that good for them either. You don't want to pass on the bad food habits that you are fighting off. If you are uncomfortable with depriving your children of their favorite treats, try setting aside a special kitchen drawer or cabinet that is just for their foods. Don't allow yourself to raid and replace the goodies you set aside for them.

If you want to keep a favorite indulgence on hand, such as chocolates or cookies, but you and perhaps the rest of your family need some help in self-control, try this tactic. Keep cookies, candy, chocolates, and sliced single-serving cakes and pastries in the freezer. Make it a requirement that you take out only one at a time, and allow it to thaw at room temperature before you eat it. That think-before-you-eat delay will help keep you from sticking an extra two or three hundred calories in your mouth!

If you are alone and bored and there is something in the house that you just cannot stay away from—leftover dessert or an opened bag of goodies—just throw it out! Right away! We were all taught to not to waste food, but when the food in question is high-fat, high-sugar, or additive-laden, it is of poor nutritional value and not needed in our well-fed society. You will be amazed at how relieved you feel after emptying the bag of cookies into the garbage can or flushing the rest of the ice cream down the sink with hot water. The little twinge of guilt you might feel about wasting food doesn't compare to the guilt you would inevitably feel if you ate the stuff.

In binge-proofing your house, try to keep all food put away in the kitchen out of sight, with perhaps only a bowl of fruit to invite snacking. Whenever it is time for a meal or a snack, the following guidelines should help you control mindless overconsumption:

- Never eat out of the package, container, or bowl. Put all food on plates, single-serving size. Go back for seconds if necessary and again put the food on the plate before eating.

- Eat only when seated at the table. Don't allow yourself to eat in the kitchen, on the sofa, or in bed.
- Give your food your full attention. Don't eat while cooking or watching TV. You'll lose track of your consumption, and eat more than you need or really want.

Not So SAD (or Depressed) Anymore

Light therapy is unquestionably the best treatment for seasonal affective disorder (SAD). Depending on the severity of your symptoms, you may want to invest in a light box or build one yourself if you have the skills. As suggested in chapter 4, before you spend the money, you may wish to check with a doctor to be certain your symptoms truly are SAD rather than chronic mood and eating problems that happen to be worse during a particular winter. If your symptoms are moderate or tolerable, increased exposure to natural daylight along with well-chosen carbohydrate meals may provide you with all the benefit you need. It is now well established that morning exposure to bright light is the best treatment for SAD (equal or superior to antidepressants). So you might try restructuring your day to allow you some time outside in the morning—perhaps by parking in a more distant location and walking—part of your regular commute.

A thirty-minute walk on a wintry or cloudy day can have a decided impact on improving how you feel. Even on the most overcast days, the intensity of outside light is many times greater than that of the most brightly lit room or office. You may be avoiding the outdoors during the winter out of a concern that too much exposure will dry out and age your skin. In fact, it is the hot, dry air inside our homes and offices that accounts for most of the punishment the skin suffers during the winter. You are better off turning down the temperature on your thermostat than avoiding the outdoors. You can wear a ski mask or bundle up everything but your eyes if the cold bothers you. According to a Swedish proverb, there is no bad weather, only bad clothing. Now there are so many lightweight high-tech fabrics for winter sports clothing (such as Gore-Tex, PolyPro, Polar Fleece, Thinsulate, among many others) that no one needs to shiver under bulky layers of wool sweaters and nylon jackets with polyester fill. (Assuming you are not so fashion-conscious as to care whether this season's jackets have different reflective pin striping or other minor modifications, you can often find huge discounts online for discontinued items or last year's styles.) But if the weather outside is frightful, even sitting close to a window can be beneficial.

If you tend to have ups and downs throughout the year, getting outdoors more, particularly to exercise, can be very helpful in any season, summer as well as winter. Over the past twenty years, we have all been urged to stay indoors and avoid excessive exposure to sunlight for fear of skin cancer. This is certainly a real concern, given the worldwide rise in the incidence of melanoma and other cancers of the skin. However, consistent daily or near-daily sun exposure is actually protective against malignant melanoma. It is the people who vacation at the beach but spend the rest of the year indoors who put themselves at increased risk. Only your eyes need to be exposed for you to get the mood-elevating benefits of sunlight, so cover up with loose cotton clothing if you are going to be out longer or in more direct light than usual. If glare bothers your eyes, a hat with a brim is preferable to sunglasses. Exercising outdoors is invigorating, uplifting, and healthy, provided you do avoid exposures to extreme sun, heat, or cold.

Otherwise, realize that your carbohydrate craving is your body's attempt to self-medicate a serotonin deficiency. You are very likely to be one of those who feel energized by carbohydrates and sleepy after a protein meal. If your experience bears that out, you will definitely want to select a healthy carbohydrate breakfast and lunch, plus any snacks needed to keep you going. The evening meal is likely to be the best time for you to consume protein, whether it is taken in the form of dairy products, a few ounces of meat or poultry, or a complete vegetable protein, such as beans and rice. Selecting satisfying complex carbohydrates such as pasta, rice, good bread, and potatoes (not fried), along with an assortment of fruits and vegetables, should keep you feeling better without gaining weight during the winter months. In fact, once you have learned to recognize and treat or prevent your SAD symptoms, you may find that winter is not so depressing and dreary at all!

From SAD to Glad

- Increase your exposure to natural light. Exercise outdoors, work near a window, try full-spectrum lighting.
- Follow a serotonin-enhancing diet with emphasis on complex carbohydrates, especially in the winter.
- Keep a Food-Mood-Activity Journal for your winter symptoms, noting the positive effects of foods, activities, and exercise.
- Wear sunglasses only as needed to reduce glare.

Brightening Your Moods Year Round: Light Therapy and Sleep Deprivation

Finally, there has long been a minority view among researchers that some of the many forms of nonseasonal depression might involve phase-shift disturbances of the daily serotonin-melatonin wake-sleep cycle. (Phase-shift disturbances are a common cause of sleep disorders, as discussed in chapter 2.) Several studies have detected abnormal circadian rhythms of specific hormones and immune modulators in depressed patients. Recently, Danish researchers have reported that bright light therapy is useful as a supplemental therapy for major depression (given in conjunction with antidepressant medication), although it has never been shown effective as a stand-alone therapy for non-SAD mood disorders. Although the evidence here is far from overwhelming, there is no obvious downside for people with mild to moderate depression to seek more or better bright light exposure. Phase-shift disturbances are more likely to be present if the individual also has problems with sleep (insomnia or oversleeping), is troubled more by low energy and fatigue than by tearfulness or negativity, and has daily mood cycles (for example, worse in the morning, better at night).

Have you ever been roused out of bed at, say, 4 A.M. for an early flight, or stayed up all night for some reason or another, and then been surprised to find that you actually felt pretty good—alert, cheerful, productive—for the rest of the day? Well, you were on to something! On a do-it-yourself level, sleep deprivation fairly reliably, though temporarily, lifts the mood of depressed patients. The classic studies showing efficacy were all-nighters plus—total sleep deprivation for about thirty-six hours. Subsequent studies established that partial sleep deprivation—a normal bedtime with about four hours of sleep, then staying awake until the next night—is also effective as a very rapid, though short-lived treatment for depression. One small study reported achieving a more durable benefit with a program of total sleep deprivation on day one, sleep from 5 P.M. to midnight on day two, then postponing sleep time an hour each night until the individual was back on a normal sleep schedule. Sleep deprivation followed by some other form of therapy can be effective in sustaining improved moods. People with mild-to-moderate depressive symptoms who would like to avoid medication could try combining partial sleep deprivation and bright light therapy. This should be obvious (but I had better state it anyway): If you try sleep deprivation, don't operate a car or other dangerous machinery when you are seriously behind on sleep.

12

∿

Putting It All Together— Making It Work

Every person is unique in mood and in behavior, in health and in illness. Your biochemistry is as distinctively you as your face and your personality. One-size-fits-all solutions make poor sense and poor self-care approaches. This chapter will guide you in pulling together the information and recommendations in this book and tailoring them to create a practical and rewarding nutrition and activity program that will produce optimal results for you.

Personal preferences obviously come first. Any self-care plan that requires you to accept restrictive or unpleasant food and exercise requirements is simply not going to work. Since a majority of readers will have some mood and impulse control problems, a program that involves self-denial is likely to make the problem much worse. For this reason, chapters 9 and 10 have offered a broad menu of choices, going by the philosophy that even a little change is a lot more than no change! If you have tended to be anxious, overweight, and sedentary, don't push yourself to work out every day and dine on broccoli and brown rice. Instead, start by choosing familiar, comforting foods—pasta with a hearty tomato sauce or good-quality breads and muffins. Start with walking more on nice days and practicing deep breathing, plus simple repetitive flexibility exercises, such as those described in chapter 10. Make your goal a positive one—feeling better and having more energy. Don't focus on negatives such as being overweight until you feel more positive and motivated.

The specific problems you are targeting also make a difference. Migraine sufferers need to be on the alert for specific foods, behavior, or activities that may be triggering headaches. People with SAD may need only a program that gets them through the cold and dreary months of winter. People with overcharged, hyperalert anxiety symptoms will have different mood-elevating goals and may respond differently to specific foods and exercises than people who are more often troubled by feeling low, fatigued, and listless. *Individual differences in body and brain chemistry need first to be respected and explored.* As chapter 9 explained, high-carbohydrate foods will make some people calm, even sleepy, while others will be energized by them. The first step is to monitor and record how your mood and behavior are affected by specific foods, events, and activities.

Your Daily Food-Mood-Activity Journal

To find out how foods, activities, and environmental factors affect you, you need to set up a log or journal in which you record the foods you eat, your activities (and inactivities!), and how they affect your mood and functioning over the next two or three hours; you need to repeat this every time you eat or exercise. Recording these basic, often overlooked details may well be filled with surprises and insights for you. You will see, first of all, how you really do eat day in and day out. In the pressure and the rush, we eat what's there—and neglect fundamental nutritional goals, like keeping the fat content below 30 percent, or having five servings of fruits and vegetables per day. You will see how often you break your own little rules, like "just one glass of wine before dinner." Or how often you eat automatically, gobbling down appetizers at a party or chips in front of the TV. More importantly, you'll see that the foods and drinks you crave or overeat when your mood is low may be bringing it still lower. You will also see how much you are influenced by weather, time of day, and other factors, and how knowing your low-mood or high-pain times will help you to predict and control your symptoms.

The journal also serves as your prove-it-to-yourself assurance that food choices and activities do have a dramatic impact on how you feel, function, and behave.

Your journal should be not much more than a simple log of what you eat, what you do, and how it affects your target issues—whether that's your mood state, chronic pain, binge eating, drinking, or other impulse control problems. A good guideline is to keep it so brief and businesslike that you would not be embarrassed to share it with a family member, friend, or doctor if you wanted them to see what you had learned from keeping your daily food-mood-activity records. A suggested format is provided at the end of the chapter.

You may also want to keep a separate motivational journal where you practice positive self-talk, and explore what you have learned about yourself and about the factors that relieve or intensify your serotonin-related symptoms.

Body and Mind Awareness

Keeping a daily Food-Mood-Activity Journal is just about guaranteed to give you some surprises. We tend to assume that the foods we most desire make us feel good—why else would we eat them? In fact, the cheeseburger and fries you have for lunch may taste good going down, yet when you track your mood and energy over the next few hours, you discover that the high-fat food really leaves you feeling sluggish, and you do not function at your best. Similarly, the pleasure of eating a donut or candy bar may trigger a crash a few hours later, when you become irritable, weak, or shaky. Does coffee really make you more alert, more focused? Or does it irritate your stomach and make you jittery? The first drink of the evening really did relax you, but the second or third one made you groggy, or brought on a slight tension headache. Once you document for yourself how foods affect your moods, you may find it easier to break eating habits that give five minutes of gratification in exchange for several hours of physical and mental discomfort.

Be sure to note the *quantities* of food you consume. Although we so easily forget this simple but important fact (particularly when there is too much food on our plate and we're bored, distracted, or depressed), the quantity of food eaten has a very obvious effect on mood and energy. An afternoon energy sag or performance decline can be traced to a large (1,000 calorie) lunch, which will not occur with a 300-calorie balanced lunch. Although it can be unpleasant to be hungry, it does keep you alert. If you are drowsy and unproductive by mid to late afternoon, experiment with having a smaller lunch, then a small fruit-and-crackers type snack when your hunger returns.

The pharmaceutical companies would like us to believe otherwise, but heartburn, gastroesophageal reflux (GERD), nausea, and upset stomach are not inevitable aspects of the human condition. When you have symptoms of indigestion in the hour or so after a meal, all those serotonin receptors in the gut and the brain stem are trying to send you an important message: "Nasty! Spoiled! Too greasy! Too much! Don't do it again!" Be sure and note down any indigestion or gastric upset in your Food-Mood-Activity Journal. Try to determine whether food quality or quantity was responsible for your symptoms. Then listen to your gut and don't do it again.

Keep the same careful mood records for choice of activity. When you come home from work feeling stressed, depressed, or deprived, exercise can seem like just another part of the daily burden of "doing what you're supposed to do, not what you want to do." You change clothes and slump on the sofa with a food or alcohol treat. If your mood is okay and your day was physically active, that may be just what you need. However, inactivity will ultimately bring a low mood lower. If you have sleeping problems, inactivity and overeating or drinking will make them worse. Get yourself to take an evening stroll or bicycle ride just once or twice for the sake of comparison. Check how you feel on getting up the next morning, as well as how you feel and function for the rest of the evening.

Most people just are not that aware of how their body and mind feel from moment to moment, unless something is wrong. Little fluctuations in our mood, in our physical comfort and vitality, tend to go unnoticed, pushed below the threshold of awareness by other concerns. We may not notice that our mood has slowly shifted up or down until the change is obvious to ourselves or others. We may gage our body's health and well-being only in negative terms: by a sudden flare-up of pain or by getting on the bathroom scale. Your journal will help you become aware of the subtle shifts in feeling and energy we go through every day. Awareness is step one to achieving control.

Some individuals can have rapid, extreme shifts in mood and energy. A few have impulses so sudden and powerful that they act on them before they are even aware. For the majority of us, moods and impulses build slowly. A shift in mood or a desire for a high-calorie snack starts below the threshold of awareness and then grows, snowballs, to dominate consciousness and displace competing feelings and ideas. The key to managing mood shifts and eating and other impulses is to detect them quickly and defeat them before they mushroom out of control, through selecting an enjoyable substitute or a distracting activity.

Set Short-Term Goals

Goal 1: Find Out for Yourself

As you begin to design and follow your own mood, pain, and impulse-control program, try setting simple, concrete goals on a weekly or monthly basis. Goal number one should be simply learning more about how foods and activities affect you. Don't attempt to change or reverse your habits and lifestyle, or make rules for yourself, until you have explored how your usual ways of managing your days might be helping or hurting you. Of course, you know you should eat more fruits and vegetables and less ice cream and chips. Of course, you know you should get more exercise. But, bottom line, we are going to do the things we perceive as pleasurable and mood enhancing, while avoiding everything we perceive as unenjoyable and burdensome. The important word here is "perceive." Because we focus on the moment, we often miss the connection between what we do right now and how we feel two to six hours later, or the next day. We may see it when the results of eating and drinking much too much are dramatic—an upset stomach or a hangover. We can overlook the cause-and-effect connection when what we experience is a relatively subtle dip in physical well-being and good spirits that takes a few hours to develop.

As you begin to log how you feel with your usual eating and activity routine, start experimenting in small, easy-to-manage ways. Take that walk and record how you feel afterward. Substitute a different afternoon snack and see if you might get better mood and appetite control. You are not yet on a diet or exercise plan. You are innovating and learning about what feels good for you. Allow at least a month of daily recording and experimenting without setting rules or restrictions.

At the end of the month, list the foods and activities that produced the best results for you, versus those that seemed to bring on symptoms. You will want to keep on checking and recording in the coming months, since you may well have seasonal variations, as well as events and changes in your life that will inevitably play a part in how you feel. Use these preliminary results to see if you can make some generalizations about how basic dietary factors—fat, sugar, caffeine, alcohol, protein, and carbohydrates—affect how you feel and function. Refer back to the information in chapters 8 and 9 to help you generalize and identify other feel-good foods.

Try to identify how different physical activities have positively affected you over the month—calming anxiety, lifting mood and energy, curbing appetite, or reducing pain. Specify the impact on mood, energy, pain, and impulse control of such categories of activity as: (*a*) an aerobic workout, (*b*) milder cardiovascular exercise, like walking or leisurely bicycling, (*c*) repetitive movement exercises as described in chapter 10, (*d*) hobbies and crafts such as knitting or woodworking, and (*e*) deep breathing and relaxation techniques. Notice whether time of day makes a difference in the effects. Use the information and lists provided in chapter 10 to develop other ideas for serotonin-enhancing activities. If you have been inactive, plan to walk or do repetitive movement exercises at or shortly before the times of day when you usually droop. For example, you can do the exercises when you wake up, get out at noon for walking and shopping, then spend some time on an enjoyable hobby in the evening. When you start to feel better, substitute an aerobic workout for one of those activities and discover the mood-elevating and pain-relieving effects of working your heart, lungs, and muscles.

Goal 2: Feel Better

For the next month of your record-keeping, you still don't want to set requirements, such as "knock it off with the donuts" or "exercise three hours per week." Instead, define goal 2 in positive terms simply as "feeling better." If you have an appetite or other impulse control problem, rate your days according to your mood and energy state rather than your eating, drinking, or spending behavior. At this point, you don't want to judge yourself on what you do, simply on how you feel. Give each day a one- to four-star rating, based entirely on how you felt—your mood and energy level—over the course of the day. Provided you are not doing anything absurdly unhealthy or risky, focus simply on increasing the number of three-star and four-star days in your month. Continue to observe and record how foods and activities influence how you feel.

During this phase, you should work as needed on developing positive self-talk techniques, as described in chapter 11. Mild serotonin-related problems can often be relieved simply by attention to the selection and timing of serotonin-enhancing foods and activities. For those who have long-standing problems with mood or negativity, attention to changing mental habits, as well as lifestyle, can be extremely helpful. For example, perhaps you continually beat up on yourself about your weight or obsess over every little mistake you make. Enhancing your serotonin activity won't undo negative thinking all by itself. Use a second, motivational journal to develop positive ways of thinking about yourself and your life. If you are annoyed about something you did on a particular day, such as eating or drinking too much, work on it in your motivational journal. Don't let it influence how many stars you give yourself in your Food-Mood-Activity Journal.

Goal 2 should require a minimum of a month. You may find that focusing on feeling good and identifying the foods and activities needed to improve mood and relieve pain will naturally lead you to making healthier choices for yourself. If you have addictions and cravings that will take more concentrated effort to curb, don't take them on until you have worked yourself up to a calendar of mostly three- and four-star days. Feeling energetic, upbeat, and in control are essential prerequisites to working on problem areas that will make demands on your capacity for self-restraint and self-denial and your ability to reverse well-established habits.

Goal 3: Change Unhealthy Habits

Goal 3, then, should be gaining better control over any unhealthy habits still remaining. Continue to use your Food-Mood-Activity Journal to motivate you and help you assess your progress. This is a more difficult goal that has the potential to bring your mood down through feelings of deprivation or guilt and frustration over any failures, real or imagined. For this reason, use a second progress-marking system. Continue to award yourself stars based on how you feel. Give yourself a check mark for every time you successfully curb a habit or impulse that troubles you.

If you have problems meeting the specifics of your goal, reexamine it. Is it a goal that truly has to do with health and well-being, or is it just cosmetic? For example, if your goal is "curb my bingeing and purging" or "stop blowing money whenever I'm blue," those are important concerns to work on. If, on the other hand, your focus is "lose twenty pounds" or "get rid of this awful cellulite," those may not be either realistic or worthwhile goals to pursue. Avoid setting difficult-to-meet cosmetic goals that will only make you feel bad when you fail.

If you have difficulty curbing a food or alcohol impulse, experiment with two different strategies. Control your access to or ration your supply of a beloved food, using one of the techniques described in chapter 11. For example, if you love chocolate but have not been able to control how much of it you eat, keep it out of your home and your office. If you have to make a separate trip for it, you will eat less. If there is still candy beckoning you from coworkers' desks or snack machines, try telling yourself "I deserve only the best." Reward yourself for avoiding the cheap stuff with a weekly gift to yourself of a few pieces or a quarter pound of high-quality chocolate from a gourmet shop.

Record the results of your rationing efforts in your Food-Mood-Activity Journal. If you find you still lose control, or simply feel too many pangs of longing and craving, try a cold turkey withdrawal. If your weakness is chocolate or other sweets, try eliminating all refined sugar and artificial sweeteners from your diet for at least a month, along with foods that contain large amounts of honey or molasses. If you crave high-fat foods, cut the fat content in your diet by eliminating fried foods and relying on skim or low-fat dairy products. The craving will steadily diminish and may disappear altogether. You may find that you can't even tolerate high-sugar or high-fat foods once you have withdrawn them from your diet.

Out with the Old Habits, In with the New

We all know that alcohol, nicotine, and caffeine are addictive. Attempting to cut down or do without is punished by irritability, pain, fatigue, poor concentration, and other mental and physical symptoms, depending on the severity of the habit. These substances are physically addicting: changes take place in specific neurotransmitter systems as the brain becomes accustomed to its daily hit of the addictive substance. They are also psychologically or situationally addictive. We develop a mental and emotional dependence on having a cigarette or a drink in specific situations or settings, such as after dinner. Many people are able to grit their teeth and bear the pain and mood changes of cutting back or quitting cold turkey. Ultimately, they may not be able to sustain it because of the psychological addiction. They can't concentrate on their work without a cup of coffee before them at all times, or they can't feel comfortable in a social setting without a cigarette or a drink.

Similarly, we become psychologically or situationally addicted to our eating habits and especially to high-fat and high-sugar foods. There are no jelly donut receptors that trigger a physical addiction to sweet, gooey pastries. Nonetheless, if you regularly have some high-calorie, low-nutrition treat in the morning or as an afternoon snack, you may find it very hard to do without it. Fighting the impulse can interfere with your concentration, and you may become acutely aware of any emotional or physical discomfort that you are accustomed to medicating with food.

Offer your habit a substitute pleasure. If you go for sweets, have a banana or a packet of raisins instead. You will get a healthier, more sustained energy boost, and you won't feel drugged or groggy from eating a snack with too much fat. Once your taste for sweets adjusts to accepting the high-sugar fruits, try giving yourself a lower-calorie higher-fiber fruit treat, an apple, orange, peach, or grapefruit. Foods that take a little time to eat, like an apple or an orange, can be more satisfying as serotonin-enhancing snacks. Remember that chewing increases serotonin system activity.

Our daily habits and routine have great powers for reinforcing themselves. Have you ever deliberately left the house without your wallet or handbag and found yourself very uncomfortable without it, repeatedly patting your pocket or reaching for the bag? Or rearranged your desk, then continued to look for items in their old places for weeks afterward? We have very strong impulses to keep doing whatever we have been doing for a long time. Just as you learn the new locations of your desk contents, you can replace one habit with another. The afternoon candy bar gets replaced with fruit or a low-sugar, low-fat muffin. Once you have grown accustomed to your new snack, the candy bar will be sickeningly sweet.

The standard recommendation for people who have been inactive is to exercise three times a week for thirty minutes to an hour. You may get better results by doing some level of exercise on a daily basis, as close to the same time every day as practical. For example, when you get up in the morning, try doing some simple flexibility exercises, as described in chapter 10. Keep them short and simple so they seem more like an elaborate yawn-and-stretch rather than a burdensome exercise requirement. As they start to become a pleasant, almost automatic habit, you can make them a little more vigorous. In time, they will do the job of waking you up much better than a cup of coffee.

If you don't usually socialize or do business at lunch, use the noon hour to walk, just saving fifteen minutes at the end of your lunch break for a light carbohydrate lunch, as suggested in chapter 10. You will eat less and feel more refreshed and alert. If there is a gym or fitness club near your home or near your office, consider joining. Many have trial memberships or memberships on a month-to-month basis. Start by doing only the things you find enjoyable or at least neutral, such as swimming or walking on a treadmill. Or just go to sit in the sauna. Establish a regular routine of showing up at the gym and enjoying the social contact with other members. Once going to the gym is a habit you can begin to put more pressure on yourself to work at it.

Setting Up Your Food-Mood-Activity Journal

The best and easiest-to-manage format is that of a daily planner or weekly calendar that gives a page to each day, with adequate fill-in space next to the daytime hours. Record all your foods and activities plus any events and environmental factors that might have affected you. You can indicate mood, energy, and other target symptoms using this scale:

at my worst	bad/poor	mildly negative	neutral	mildly positive	good	at my best
−3	−2	−1	0	1	2	3

Try to record both how you feel at the time of a snack, meal or activity, and then record your mood, energy, and other symptoms about an hour or two later, or whenever you notice a shift up or down in how you function and feel.

Date:_____

7 A.M.: Wake-up: energy −2, mood 0

8 A.M.: orange juice, bran muffin—energy 0, mood 0

9 A.M.: Parked in cheap lot & walked, 10 min.—energy 1, mood 1

10 A.M.: energy 1, mood 1

11 A.M.: same

NOON: Walked for 20 min.; lunch: fresh veggie & pasta salad— energy 2, mood 2

1 P.M.: energy 3, mood 2

2 P.M.: same

3 P.M.: energy 2, mood 2

4 P.M.: energy 1, mood 2; snack: banana

5 P.M.: energy 2, mood 2

6 P.M.: commute, errands; energy 1, mood 1

7 P.M.: chicken stir-fry; energy 1, mood 3

8 P.M.: energy 1, mood 3

9 P.M.: same

10 P.M.: bedtime

OTHER
FACTORS: Cloudy, sky cleared in afternoon; very busy workday.

NOTES: Less sleepy after light lunch; banana was good pick-me-up. I wanted something with chocolate, but I actually felt better longer. Walking helped a lot, too.

Obviously, you can develop your own system for recording these simple facts and the symptoms and changes that are most of interest to you. You can add more detail if you like about how foods and activities affect you or how your moods and energy ebb and flow throughout the day. Or, you can cut it down to a few cryptic entries, such as "swim 20 laps—E3, M3," and really puzzle a curious coworker or snoopy kid!

Whenever you spot a food or activity that makes a difference in how you feel, be sure you make a note of it, literally. We all eat and drink too much and then say afterward, "I wish I hadn't." Yet, urged by our cravings and our symptoms, we overindulge again and again. If you make the effort to record the hangover effects of indulging a craving, versus the sustained positive effects of eating feel-good foods, your choice will be clearer to you. Control the craving, and get a reward later. Satisfy the craving, and get punished for it. Growing up, we learn to respect other people's property because we know we will be punished if we grab what we want. Our body tries to train us by the same methods used by parents, teachers, and playmates, but we tend to ignore the message or miss the connection. You can learn to keep away from your own cookie jar by paying more attention to the punishment your body gives you.

Talk Back to Your Skepticism, Fight Your Inertia

When you are fighting mood, self-control, or pain problems, there is an almost overwhelming urge to stick to the easy and familiar patterns. After a sleepless night or during a throbbing headache, on a gloomy day when you are stressed and burdened, you naturally want to give in to food cravings and to avoid putting out more than a just-get-by level of effort. On a good day, you might think, "I'm fine, I don't need to stick to this plan today."

Long-term improvement in how you feel, behave, and perform requires step-by-step effort. The steps are small, easy, and rewarding, but changing any habit always takes a conscious decision. If you find yourself thinking, "Nah, it can't really work," talk back to your negative attitude. Tell yourself:

1. I know eating right and being more active is good for me, even if there isn't an obvious effect on my mood, energy, self-control, or headaches. So there's bound to be *some* benefit.
2. It can't hurt; it can only help. Plus, it doesn't cost anything.
3. I can try it once or twice. If it doesn't help, at least I tried.

All of the serotonin-friendly recommendations given in this book satisfy conditions one and two. With the exception of an elimination diet to identify migraine triggers, one or two experiments with healthier food and activity choices should be enough to give you some idea of the benefits of sticking to a feel-good, serotonin-friendly lifestyle.

Selected References

Barondes, Samuel H. Thinking about Prozac. *Science* 263 (1994): 1102–1104.

Baughan, David M. Barriers to diagnosing anxiety disorders in family practice. *American Family Physician.* 52 (1995): 447–451.

Biegon, Anat. Effects of steroid hormones on the serotonergic system. *Annals of the New York Academy of Sciences* 600 (1990): 427–434.

Blundell, John E. Serotonin and the biology of feeding. *American Journal of Clinical Nutrition* 55 (1992): 155S–159S.

Blundell, John E.; Burley, V. J.; Cotton, J. R.; and Lawton, C. L. Dietary fat and the control of energy intake: Evaluating the effects of fat on meal size and postmeal satiety. *American Journal of Clinical Nutrition* 57 (1993): 772S–777S.

Blundell, John E.; Green, S.; and Burley, V. Carbohydrates and human appetite. *American Journal of Clinical Nutrition* 59 (1994): 728S–734S.

Breslau, Naomi. Migraine and major depression: a longitudinal study. *Headache* 34 (1994): 387–393.

Caspi, Avshalom; Sugden, Karen; Moffitt, Terrie E.; et al. Influence of life stress on depression: moderation by a polymorphism in the 5-HTT gene. *Science* 301 (2003): 386–389.

Charney, Dennis S.; Woods, Scott W.; Krystal, John H.; and Heninger, George R. Serotonin function and human anxiety disorders. *Annals of the New York Academy of Sciences* 600 (1990): 558–569.

Christensen, Larry, and Redig, Clare. Effect of meal composition on mood. *Behavioral Neuroscience* 107 (1993): 346–53.

Curzon, G. Serotonin and appetite. *Annals of the New York Academy of Sciences* 600 (1990): 521–531.

Dahlitz, M.; Alvarez, B.; Vignau, J.; et al. Delayed sleep phase syndrome response to melatonin. *Lancet* 337 (1991):1121–1125.

Dahlitz, M., and Parkes, J. D. Sleep paralysis. *Lancet* 341 (1993): 406–408.

Danton, William G.; Altrocci, John; Antonuccio, David; and Basta, Robert. Nondrug treatment of anxiety. *American Family Physician* 49 (1994): 161–167.

Delgado, Pedro L.; Charney, D. S.; Price, L. H.; et al. Serotonin function and the mechanism of antidepressant action. *Archives of General Psychiatry* 47 (1990): 411–418.

Driver, Helen S., and Shapiro, Colin M. Parasomnias. *British Medical Journal* 306 (1993): 921–925.

Fernstrom, John D. Dietary amino acids and brain function. *Journal of the American Dietetic Association* 94 (1994): 71–77.

Fernstrom, John D. Tryptophan, serotonin, and carbohydrate appetite: Will the real carbohydrate craver please stand up! *Journal of Nutrition* 118 (1988): 1417–1419.

Fernstrom, John D, and Wurtman, Richard J. Brain serotonin content: Physiological regulation by plasma neutral amino acids. *Science* 178 (1972): 414–416.

Fernstrom, Madelyn H., and Fernstrom, John D. Brain tryptophan concentrations and serotonin synthesis remain responsive to food consumption after the ingestion of sequential meals. *American Journal of Clinical Nutrition* 61 (1995): 312–319.

Gilbert, Paul, and Sloman, Leon (eds). *Subordination and Defeat: An Evolutionary Approach to Mood Disorders and Their Therapy*. Mahwah, N.J.: Lawrence Erlbaum Associates, 2000.

Golden, Robert N.; Gilmore, John H.; Corrigan, Mark; et al. Serotonin, suicide and aggression: Clinical studies. *Journal of Clinical Psychiatry* 51 (12 suppl) (1991): 61–69.

Golier, Julia A.; Marzuk, Peter M.; Leon, Andrew C.; et al. Low serum cholesterol level and attempted suicide. *American Journal of Psychiatry* 152 (1995): 419–423.

Goodwin, G. M.; Cowen, P. J.; Fairburn, C. G.; et al. Plasma concentrations of tryptophan and dieting. *British Medical Journal* 300 (1990): 1499–1501.

Gorzalka, Boris B.; Mendelson, Scott D.; and Watson Neil V. Serotonin receptor subtypes and sexual behavior. *Annals of the New York Academy of Sciences* 600 (1990): 435–446.

Green, S. M.; Burley, V. J.; and Blundell, J. E. Effect of fat and sucrose containing foods on the size of eating episodes and energy intake in lean males: potential for causing overconsumption. *European Journal of Clinical Nutrition* 48 (1994): 547–555.

Haimov, I.; Laudon, M.; Zisapel, N.; et al. Sleep disorders and melatonin rhythms in elderly people. *British Medical Journal* 309 (1994): 167.

Hart, Carol. Forged in St. Anthony's fire: drugs for migraine. *Modern Drug Discovery* 2 (2) (1999): 20–31.

Hart, Carol. The mysterious placebo effect. *Modern Drug Discovery* 2(4) (1999): 30–40.

Hernandez, Luis; Parada, Marco.; Baptista, Trino; et al. Hypothalamic serotonin in treatments for feeding disorders and depression as studied by brain microdialysis. *Journal of Clinical Psychiatry* 51 (12 suppl) (1991): 32–40.

Hill, A. J.; Magson, L. D.; and Blundell, J. E. Hunger and palatability: Tracking ratings of subjective experience before, during, and after the consumption of preferred and less preferred food. *Appetite* 5 (1984): 361–371.

Jacobs, Barry L. Serotonin and behavior: Emphasis on motor control. *Journal of Clinical Psychiatry* 51 (12 suppl) (1991): 17–23.

Jacobs, Barry L., and Azmitia, Efrain C. Structure and function of the brain serotonin system. *Physiological Reviews* 72 (1992): 165–215.

Jacobs, Barry L., and Fornal, Casimir A. Activity of serotonergic neurons in behaving animals. *Neuropsychopharmacology* 21 (1999): 9S–15S.

Jimerson, David C.; Lesem, Michael D.; Hegg, Arlene P.; and Brewerton, Timothy D. Serotonin in human eating disorders. *Annals of the New York Academy of Sciences* 600 (1990): 532–544.

Kaplan, Jay, et al. Demonstration of an association among dietary cholesterol, central serotonergic activity and social behavior in monkeys. *Psychosomatic Medicine* 56 (1994): 479–484.

Kawachi, I.; Sparrow, D.; Vokonas, P. S.; et al. Symptoms of anxiety and risk of coronary heart disease. *Circulation* 90 (1994): 2225–2229.

Kaye, Walter H. and Weltzin, Theodore E. Serotonin activity in anorexia and bulimia nervosa: Relationship to the modulation of feeding and mood. *Journal of Clinical Psychiatry* 51 (12 suppl) (1991): 41–48.

Khan, Arif; Khan, Shirin R.; Walens, Gary; Kolts, Russell; and Giller, Earl L. Frequency of positive studies among fixed and flexible dose antidepressant clinical trials: An analysis of the Food and Drug Administration summary basis of approval reports. *Neuropsychopharmacology* 28 (2003): 552–557.

Lader, Malcolm. Treatment of anxiety. *British Medical Journal* 309 (1994): 321–325.

LaForge, Ralph. Post-exercise euphoria: Why you feel good. *Executive Health Report* 27 (1990): 6.

Landry, Mim J. Serotonin and impulse dyscontrol: Brain chemistry involved in impulse and addictive behavior. *Behavioral Health Management* 14 (1994): 35–38.

Leibenluft, Ellen; Fiero, Patricia; and Rubinow, David R. Effects of the menstrual cycle on dependent variables in mood disorder research. *Archives of General Psychiatry* 51 (1994): 761–781.

LeMarquand, David; Pihl, Robert O.; and Benkelfat, Chawki. Serotonin and alcohol intake, abuse and dependence: Clinical evidence. *Biological Psychiatry* 36 (1994): 326–337.

Leuchter, Andrew F.; Cook, Ian A.; Witte, Elise A.; Morgan, Melinda; and Abrams, Michelle. Changes in brain function of depressed subjects during treatment with placebo. *American Journal of Psychiatry* 159 (2002): 122–129.

McElroy, Susan L. Compulsive buying: A report of 20 cases. *Journal of Clinical Psychiatry* 55 (1994): 242–248.

McSherry, James, and Ashman, George. Bulimia and sleep disturbance. *Journal of Family Practice* 30 (1990): 102–104.

Meltzer, Herbert Y. The significance of serotonin for neuropsychiatric disorders. *Journal of Clinical Psychiatry* 51 (12 suppl) (1991): 70–72.

Meltzer, Herbert Y. Role of serotonin in depression. *Annals of the New York Academy of Sciences* 600 (1990): 486–500.

Mills, Kirk C. Serotonin syndrome. *American Family Physician* 52 (1995): 1475–1483.

Moncrieff, Joanna. The antidepressant debate. *British Journal of Psychiatry*. 180 (2002): 193–194.

Moncrieff, Joanna, and Kirsch, Irving. Efficacy of antidepressants in adults. *British Medical Journal* 331 (2005): 155–157.

Morin, L.P.; Michels, K.M.; Smale L.; and Moore, R.Y. Serotonin regulation of circadian rhythmicity. *Annals of the New York Academy of Sciences* 600 (1990): 418–426.

Morris, Lois B. Social anxiety. *American Health* 14 (1995): 60–64.

Nishizawa, S.; Benkelfat, C.; Young, S. N.; et al. Differences between males and females in rates of serotonin synthesis in human brain. *Proceedings of the National Academy of Sciences* 94 (1997): 5308–5313.

Partonen, T., and Partinen, M. Light treatment for seasonal affective disorder: Theoretical considerations and clinical implications. *Acta Psychiatrica Scandinavica* 377 (suppl) (1994): 41–45.

Pihl, Robert O., and Peterson, Jordan B. Alcohol, serotonin and aggression. *Alcohol Health & Research World* 17 (1993): 113–117.

Richardson, Brian P. Serotonin and nociception. *Annals of the New York Academy of Sciences* 600 (1990): 511–520.

Rogers, P. J., and Blundell, J. E. Separating the actions of sweetness and calories: Effects of saccharin and carbohydrates on hunger and food intake in human subjects. *Physiology and Behavior* 45 (1989): 1093–1099.

Russo, Sasch; Kema, Ido P.; Fokkema, M. Rebecca; et al. Tryptophan as a link between psychopathology and somatic states. *Psychosomatic Medicine* 65 (2003): 665–671.

Schwartz, Jeffrey M.; Stoessel, Paula W.; Baxter, Lewis R. Jr.; et al. Systematic changes in cerebral glucose metabolic rate after successful behavior modification treatment of obsessive-compulsive disorder. *Archives of General Psychiatry* 53 (1996): 109–113.

Sellar, Edward M.; Higgins, Guy A.; Tomkins, Denise M.; et al. Opportunities for treatment of psychoactive substance abuse disorders with serotonergic medications. *Journal of Clinical Psychiatry* 51 (12 suppl) (1991): 49–54.

Song, G. H.; Leng, P. H.; Gwee, K. A.; Moochhala, S. M.; and Ho, K.Y. Melatonin improves abdominal pain in irritable bowel syndrome patients who have sleep disturbances: a randomised, double blind, placebo controlled study. *Gut* 54 (2005): 1402–1407.

Sourkes, Theodore L. Nutrients and the cofactors required for monoamine synthesis in nervous tissue. *Nutrition and the Brain*, vol. 3, ed. R. J. Wurtman and J. J. Wurtman. New York: Raven Press, 1979.

Steckler, Thomas, and Sahgal Arjun. The role of serotonergic-cholinergic interactions in the mediation of cognitive behaviour. *Behavioural Brain Research* 67 (1995): 165–199.

Steiger, Howard. Eating disorders and the serotonin connection: state, trait and developmental effects. *Journal of Psychiatry and Neuroscience* 29 (2004): 20–29.

Taylor, Duncan P. Serotonin agents in anxiety. *Annals of the New York Academy of Sciences* 600 (1990): 545–557.

Turner, Erick H.; Loftis, Jennifer M.; and Blackwell, Aaron D. Serotonin à la carte: supplementation with the serotonin precursor 5-hydroxytryptophan. *Pharmacology and Therapeutics* 109 (2006): 325–38.

Walley, Elizabeth J.; Beebe, Diane K.; and Clark, Jacquelyn L. Management of common anxiety disorders. *American Family Physician* 50 (1994): 1745–1756.

Wallin, M. S., and Rissanen, A. M. Food and mood: Relationship between food, serotonin and affective disorders. *Acta Psychiatrica Scandinavica* 377 (suppl) (1994): 36–40.

Wang, Qing-Ping, and Nakai, Yasumitsu. The dorsal raphe: An important nucleus in pain modulation. *Brain Research Bulletin* 34 (1994): 575–585.

Wauquer, A., and Dugovic, C. Serotonin and sleep-wakefulness. *Annals of the New York Academy of Sciences* 600 (1990): 447–520.

Wehr, Thomas A.; Duncan, Wallace C. Jr.; Sher, Leo; et al. A circadian signal of change of season in patients with seasonal affective disorder. *Archives of General Psychiatry* 58 (2001): 1108–1114.

Weltzin, Theodore E.; Fernstrom, Madelyn H.; Fernstrom, John D.; Neuberger, Shira K.; and Kaye, Walter H. Acute tryptophan depletion and increased food intake and irritability in bulimia nervosa. *American Journal of Psychiatry* 152 (1995): 1668–1671.

Weltzin, Theodore E.; Fernstrom, Madelyn H.; and Kaye, Walter H. Serotonin and bulimia nervosa. *Nutrition Reviews* 52 (1994): 399–408.

Weltzin, Theodore E.; Fernstrom, Madelyn H.; Fernstrom, John D.; et al. Acute tryptophan depletion and increased food intake and irritability in bulimia nervosa. *American Journal of Psychiatry* 152 (1995): 1668–1672.

Whittington, Craig J.; Kendall, Tim; Fonagy, Peter; Cottrell, David; Cotgrove, Andrew; Boddington, Ellen. Selective serotonin reuptake inhibitors in childhood depression: systematic review of published versus unpublished data. *Lancet* 363 (2004): 1341–5.

Young, Simon N. The use of diet and dietary components in the study of factors controlling affect in humans: a review. *Journal of Psychiatry and Neuroscience* 18 (1993): 235–44.

Zalman, Amit; Smith, Brian R.; and Gill, Kathryn. Serotonin uptake inhibitors: Effects on motivated consummatory behaviors. *Journal of Clinical Psychiatry* 51 (12 suppl) (1991): 55–60.

Zerbe, Kathryn J. *The Body Betrayed: Women, Eating Disorders and Treatment*. Washington, D.C.: American Psychiatric Press, 1993.

Index